Colour Atlas of Lacrimal Surgery

Acquisitions editor: Melanie Tait
Development editor: Zoë Youd
Production controller: Chris Jarvis
Desk editor: Jane Campbell
Cover designer: Alan Studholme

Colour Atlas of Lacrimal Surgery

Jane Olver

MB BS BSc DO FRCS FRCOphth

Consultant Ophthalmologist, Oculoplastic Surgeon
Charing Cross Hospital, London
and
Western Eye Hospital, London, UK

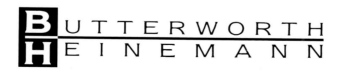

OXFORD AUCKLAND BOSTON JOHANNESBURG MELBOURNE NEW DELH

Butterworth-Heinemann
Linacre House, Jordan Hill, Oxford OX2 8DP
225 Wildwood Avenue, Woburn, MA 01801-2041
A division of Reed Educational and Professional Publishing Ltd

 A member of the Reed Elsevier plc group

First published 2002

British Library Cataloguing in Publication Data
Olver, Jane
    Colour atlas of lacrimal surgery
    1. Lacrimal apparatus – Surgery
    I. Title
    617.7'64'059

Library of Congress Cataloguing in Publication Data
Olver, Jane
    Colour atlas of lacrimal surgery/Jane Olver.
    p. ; cm.
    Includes bibliographical references and index.
    ISBN 0 7506 4486 9
    1. Lacrimal apparatus – Surgery – Atlases.   I. Title.
    [DNLM: 1. Lacrimal Apparatus – surgery – Atlases. WW 17 O52c 2002]
    RE201.O483 2002
    617.7'64059–dc21   2001043712

ISBN 0 7506 4486 9

For information on all Butterworth-Heinemann publications visit our website at www.bh.com

Composition and design by Scribe Design, Gillingham, Kent
Printed and bound in Italy

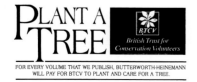

FOR EVERY VOLUME THAT WE PUBLISH, BUTTERWORTH-HEINEMANN
WILL PAY FOR BTCV TO PLANT AND CARE FOR A TREE.

Contents

Preface

Ophthalmic plastic surgery includes the management of patients with watering eyes. An ophthalmologist should be able to spot the ophthalmic causes of watering eyes, in particular work out whether there is hypersecretion, an eyelid cause or lacrimal drainage system block. As a consultant doing ophthalmic plastic surgery, I found that I had to teach lacrimal surgery to the trainees, and this book arose out of that teaching.

The aim of this book is to provide a sound basis for trainees and practitioners in lacrimal surgery. This includes the relevant anatomy needed for external and endonasal approach dacryocystorhinostomy, a systematic approach to the lacrimal assessment, and illustrated basic eyelid and lacrimal surgical techniques. I have included particulars of what is happening 'out of view', i.e. inside the nose, which until recently, for many of us, was just a dark hole. This book should help you to understand lacrimal surgery better, and encourage you to try out new techniques or improve on current ones. I would recommend that the interested reader attend endonasal dacryocystorhinostomy courses, use a nasal endoscope regularly in clinic, and try a transcanalicular diagnostic probe. The latter is revealing yet another world within the lacrimal system, which is likely to have an impact on lacrimal surgery in the future.

In basic terms, lacrimal surgery is a combination of carpentry and plumbing; operating on the eyelids and re-boring the lacrimal drainage system. It is a very practical subject, which requires a common sense approach, yet all the time maintaining the highest possible quality of craftmanship.

Patients with watering eyes don't lose their sight, but they do suffer severe functional problems from blurring, soreness and stickiness, which can be helped, especially in the frail elderly. It is worthwhile looking after this group of patients, as the results of lacrimal surgery are good and the patient's quality of life improved.

JMO 2001

Acknowledgements

I am grateful to my past Oculoplastic Fellows Chris Barras and Lorraine Cassidy, Rachel Michel (proof reader), staff of the Medical Illustration Group at the Chelsea and Westminster Hospital, Ian Mackay (otolaryngologist), and the many ophthalmic trainees who helped form this book by asking questions and taking surgical photographs. Professor Gordon Ruskell, Bijan Beigi, Raman Malhotra, Ric Caeser, Sally Webber and Robert McLaren all deserve special thanks for reading through the chapters and providing advice, as do Caroline Makepeace from Butterworth-Heinemann for taking on this project, and Ian Mulligan for his patient advice. I would like to thank Ron Knight for his help with the artwork.

CHAPTER 1

Anatomy and Physiology of the Lacrimal System

In this chapter, the anatomy is subdivided into soft tissues and osteology. Understanding both is essential for lacrimal surgeons.

Part A   *Anatomy of the lacrimal system*

Part B   *Physiology of the lacrimal system*

Part A: Anatomy of the lacrimal system

The eyelids are important in the distribution, collection and drainage of tears; malposition or dysfunction will result in a watering eye. The relations of the lacrimal sac and nasolacrimal duct to the structures of the lateral nasal wall and the ethmoid sinus are important during dacryocystorhinostomy, whether done via the external or endonasal route.

Review of the tear route

Tear secretion: Tears are produced by the lacrimal gland and accessory lacrimal tissues, the glands of Krause and Wolfring.

Tear distribution: Eyelid blinking distributes the tears over the eye and propels the tear meniscus along the eyelid margin.

Tear collection: The tears enter the puncta at the medial ends of the eyelids, passing into the upper and lower canaliculi and through the common canaliculus into the lacrimal sac. The puncta and canaliculi are regarded as the upper lacrimal drainage system.

Tear drainage: The tears drain from the lacrimal sac into the nasolacrimal duct and, through its lower opening beneath the inferior turbinate, onto the floor of the nose. The tears then trickle along the floor and into the throat. The sac and nasolacrimal duct are regarded as the lower lacrimal drainage system (Figure 1.1).

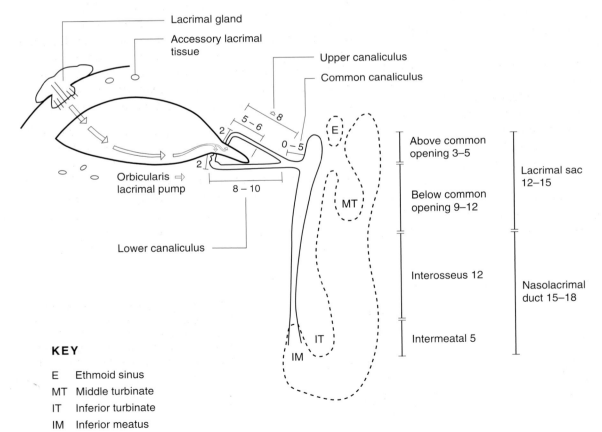

Figure 1.1

Lacrimal system – shapes and sizes.

Lacrimal gland

Accessory lacrimal tissue

Upper canaliculus

Common canaliculus

5 – 6   △8

2

0 – 5

E

2

Orbicularis ⇨ lacrimal pump

8 – 10

Above common opening 3–5

Below common opening 9–12

Lacrimal sac 12–15

MT

Lower canaliculus

Interosseus 12

Nasolacrimal duct 15–18

Intermeatal 5

IT

IM

KEY

E   Ethmoid sinus

MT   Middle turbinate

IT   Inferior turbinate

IM   Inferior meatus

All dimensions in millimetres

I. Soft tissue

There are six important soft tissues:

1. Lacrimal gland
2. Eyelids – in particular, the orbicularis at the medial canthus
3. Puncta and canaliculi – in particular, the acute angle of entry of the common canaliculus into the lacrimal sac
4. Lacrimal sac – its location, relations and surgical approaches
5. Nasolacrimal duct – its structure, relations and opening into the nose
6. Nose – lateral nasal wall and adjacent sinuses.

Lacrimal gland

The lacrimal gland lies in a fossa in the frontal bone in the antero-superior lateral orbit. The gland measures approximately 20 × 15 mm, and is flattened to approximately 5 mm. There is a main orbital lobe (superior) and smaller palpebral lobe, divided by fibrous extensions from Whitnall's ligament, the levator aponeurosis and its lateral horn. The palpebral lobe may prolapse through a thinned orbital septum with age and be visible as a subtle supero-lateral eyelid swelling. Normally 10–12 lacrimal ductules open into the supero-lateral conjunctival fornix, where they are easily identified on biomicroscopy when topical fluorescein 2% is instilled directly over the supero-lateral conjunctival fornix. The lacrimal ductules occasionally form individual cysts – dacryocoeles – which are treated by marsupialization (using an operating microscope). The accessory lacrimal glands of Krause and of Wolfring are found mainly in the upper conjunctival fornix and tarsal conjunctiva respectively. At eyelid surgery, for instance forming a lateral tarsal strip, we also identify small islands of accessory lacrimal tissue below the lateral canthal tendon.

Eyelids and orbiculari

The eyelids are responsible for tear distribution, and the orbicularis medial heads enveloping the lacrimal sac assist tear drainage.

External appearance

The upper eyelid margin normally lies 1–2 mm below the superior corneal limbus, and the lower eyelid margin level with the inferior corneal limbus. Adult vertical palpebral apertures measure 7–11 mm. The upper margin reflex distance (MRD) ranges from 2–5 mm. The lower MRD is usually 5 mm, but will reach 7–8 mm with ageing eyelid laxity and other causes of lower scleral show, including congenital malar hypoplasia, thyroid eye disease and cicatricial ectropion. With ageing eyelid changes, the upper MRD reduces and the lower MRD increases. The medial canthi are usually 1–2 mm lower than the lateral canthi; this is often lost in the ageing face, where the lateral canthi droop (Figure 1.2).

The lacrimal puncta lie at the medial ends of the eyelids, approximately 6 mm from the medial canthal angle. They are just on the posterior aspect of the eyelid margin, where they face towards the 'lacrimal lake'. With increasing age, the puncta can face upwards (and may still be effective) or slightly outwards (becoming less effective). Mild punctal eversion represents early ectropion.

Comparison of eyelid positions in young and elderly

Young adult

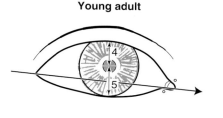

Upper MRD 4 mm
Lower MRD 5 mm

Ageing adult

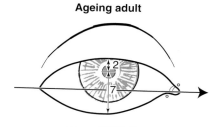

Upper MRD 2 mm
Lower MRD 7 mm

Figure 1.2

MRD = margin reflex distance in mm. The overall palpebral aperture is similar in the young and elderly, but there is relative upper eyelid ptosis and lower eyelid sag and the lateral canthus drops with ageing.

Eyelid lamellae

There are anterior and posterior lamellae, divided by a 'grey' line visible on the eyelid margin. It is useful to recognize a middle lamella.

The anterior lamellar layers consist of:
● Thin skin; thin loose connective tissue
● Orbicularis oculi muscle and retro-orbicularis 'space', which contains loose connective tissue, nerves and blood vessels; the levator aponeurosis (upper eyelid) and capsulopalpebral fascia (lower eyelid) from the middle lamellae reach this space.

The middle lamella in the upper eyelid consists of:
● Levator aponeurosis and muscle
● Muller's superior tarsal muscle
● Pre-aponeurotic fat pad.

The middle lamella in the lower eyelid consists of:
● Capsulopalpebral fascia, smooth muscle equivalent to Muller's superior tarsal muscle
● Pre-capsulopalpebral fascia fat pad.

The posterior lamella consists of:
● Tarsal plate
● Conjunctiva (Figure 1.3).

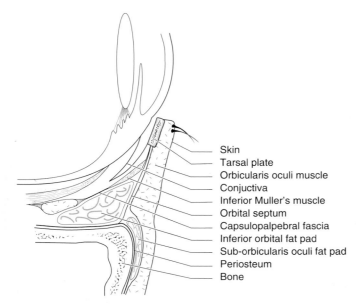

Figure 1.3
Cross-section of normal anatomy.

Skin
Tarsal plate
Orbicularis oculi muscle
Conjuctiva
Inferior Muller's muscle
Orbital septum
Capsulopalpebral fascia
Inferior orbital fat pad
Sub-orbicularis oculi fat pad
Periosteum
Bone

With ageing, soft tissue involutional changes cause horizontal eyelid laxity (HEL), orbicularis descent and orbital septal attenuation with prolapse of orbital fat forwards over the orbital rim onto the cheek. Signs of mid-face ptosis include eyelid sag and fat bulges (bags under the eyes or malar bags) and malar fold descent. The HEL and orbicularis descent weaken the lacrimal pump function of the lower eyelid and contribute to epiphora (Figure 1.4).

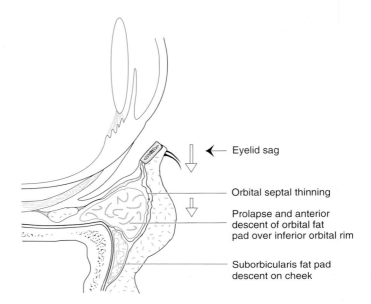

Eyelid sag

Orbital septal thinning

Prolapse and anterior descent of orbital fat pad over inferior orbital rim

Suborbicularis fat pad descent on cheek

Figure 1.4
Cross-section showing effect of ageing.

Orbicularis oculi muscle

The striated orbicularis oculi muscle is innervated by the facial nerve (CNVII) and is a protractor, which closes the eyelids. There are two distinguishable portions:

1. The orbital portion
2. The palpebral portion, which has preseptal and pretarsal parts.

The insertions of the orbicularis at the medial canthus around the lacrimal sac are called heads. The medial heads are an important part of the lacrimal system; therefore the area around the medial canthus is called the lacrimal area (LA) (Figure 1.5).

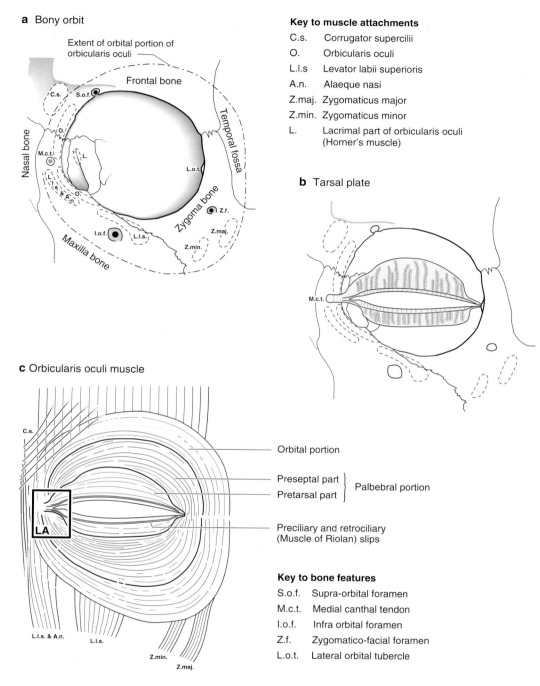

a Bony orbit

Extent of orbital portion of
orbicularis oculi

Frontal bone

Temporal fossa

Nasal bone

Zygoma bone

Maxilla bone

C.s.
S.o.f.
O.
M.c.t.
L.
L.o.t.
L & S & A.s.
O.
Z.f.
I.o.f.
L.l.s.
Z.maj.
Z.min.

Key to muscle attachments

C.s.   Corrugator supercilii

O.   Orbicularis oculi

L.l.s   Levator labii superioris

A.n.   Alaeque nasi

Z.maj. Zygomaticus major

Z.min. Zygomaticus minor

L.   Lacrimal part of orbicularis oculi
        (Horner's muscle)

b Tarsal plate

M.c.t.

c Orbicularis oculi muscle

C.s.

LA

L.l.s & A.n.
L.l.s.
Z.min.
Z.maj.

Orbital portion

Preseptal part ⎫
               ⎬ Palbebral portion
Pretarsal part ⎭

Preciliary and retrociliary
(Muscle of Riolan) slips

Key to bone features

S.o.f. Supra-orbital foramen

M.c.t. Medial canthal tendon

I.o.f. Infra orbital foramen

Z.f.   Zygomatico-facial foramen

L.o.t. Lateral orbital tubercle

Figure 1.5

Left orbit showing muscle and
tarsal plate attachments.

a) Three bones form the
    orbital rims and have the
    muscle attachments.

b) Tarsal plate is attached to
    the ascending process of
    the maxilla medially
    (outside the orbit) and to
    the lateral orbital tubercle
    laterally (inside the orbit).

c) The lacrimal area (box LA)
    is an important area with
    complicated anatomy.

Orbital portion

The orbital portion is the outermost flat sheet of
orbicularis at the edge of the orbit, overlying the frontal,
zygomatic and maxillary bones. It interdigitates with the
frontalis, corrugator supercilii and procerus muscles
superiorly, and the levator labii superioris alaeque nasi
and zygomaticus muscles inferiorly (mimetic muscles of
the face). The orbital portion is only slightly related to
the LA by a few fibres to the anterior border of the
lacrimal fossa (the anterior lacrimal crest on the frontal
process of the maxilla) above the medial canthal tendon.

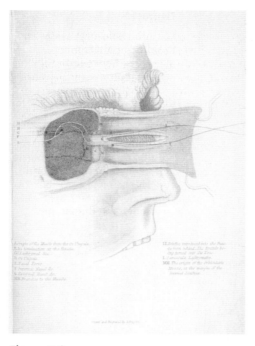

Figure 1.6

Horner's muscle. Original drawing from *Description of a Small Muscle at the Internal Commissure of the Eyelids*, by W. E. Horner, published in 1823. With permission from the Royal Society of Medicine.

Palpebral portion orbicularis

The palpebral portion of orbicularis oculi is more complex. Its attachments around the lacrimal sac form an integral part of the LA. Its preseptal and pretarsal parts lie anterior to the orbital septum and tarsus respectively. In 1961, Jones demonstrated the insertion of the superficial and deep heads around the lacrimal sac and into the posterior lacrimal crest. The deep heads of the pretarsal orbicularis are known as Horner's muscle, which is part of the lacrimal pump. Horner originally described this muscle in 1823 (Figure 1.6).

The preseptal part of the palpebral orbicularis

Circumferential preseptal fibres from the orbital septum interdigitate at the lateral commissure and contribute to the LA medially. Superficial heads insert into the medial canthal tendon. Deep heads insert into the fascia on the dome of the lacrimal sac and into the upper part of the posterior lacrimal crest (on the lacrimal bone) above the insertion of Horner's muscle. A few preseptal fibres insert below Horner's muscle.

The pretarsal part of the palpebral orbicularis

The main bulk of the pretarsal orbicularis consists of circumferential fibres in front of the superior and inferior tarsal plates. Laterally this has a loose superficial origin in the horizontal raphe and a firmer deep origin from the orbital tubercle (lateral canthal tendon) laterally. It has strong attachments medially, both to the anterior and posterior lacrimal crests, by its superficial and deep heads.

The pretarsal orbicularis also includes two small muscle slips, the marginal preciliary and retrociliary muscles (muscle of Riolan).

The marginal preciliary muscle slips are in the border of each eyelid beneath the lash roots, running between the lateral and medial commissures. Medially, anterior slips pass to the superficial part of the medial canthal tendon and posterior slips insert into Horner's muscle close to the posterior lacrimal crest. It is closely related to the muscle of Riolan and is regarded as part of it by some anatomists.

The marginal retrociliary muscle (muscle of Riolan) is a superficial part of orbicularis, which forms the appearance of the grey line on the eyelid margin. It is a 1.5 mm high × 1 mm thick slip of muscle situated adjacent to the lid margin, just behind the lash roots and closely related to the meibomian orifice openings. Its fibres interdigitate with the marginal preciliary fibres at the lateral commissure. Medially it also has fibres to the posterior lacrimal crest above and below the attachment of Horner's muscle.

Lacrimal area (LA) and Horner's muscle

The LA is between the puncta and the MCT attachment to the maxilla. The superficial and deep heads of the two palpebral parts (preseptal and pretarsal) of orbicularis, described above, surround the canaliculi and lacrimal sac. These muscle heads are fixed strongly to the bone, and therefore on blinking the eyelids are pulled medially and posteriorly. The muscle contraction propels the tear meniscus along the lower lid and compresses the canaliculi and dilates the lacrimal sac (lacrimal pump function according to Jones). Horner's muscle (deep pretarsal heads) arises from a 7–9 mm insertion along the upper part of the posterior lacrimal crest and the posterior lacrimal fascia. It bifurcates posterior to the caruncle and passes posterior to the canaliculi to the medial end of the superior and inferior tarsal plates

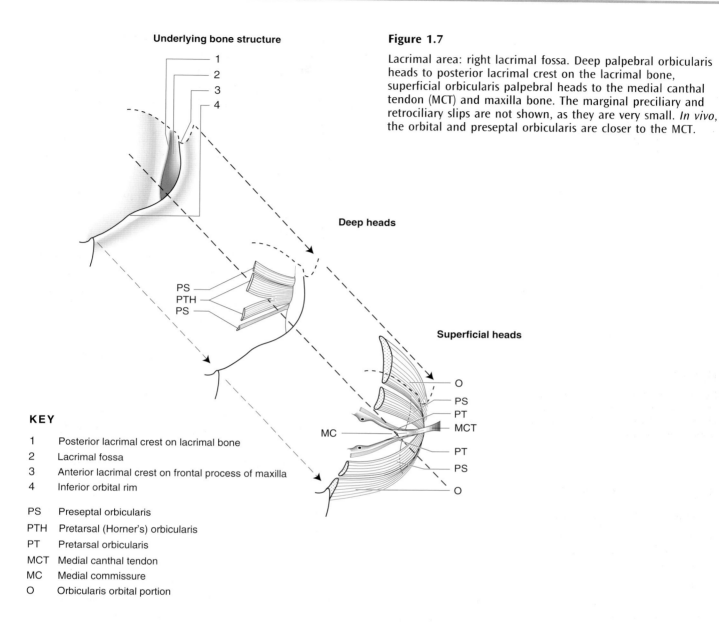

Underlying bone structure

Figure 1.7

Lacrimal area: right lacrimal fossa. Deep palpebral orbicularis heads to posterior lacrimal crest on the lacrimal bone, superficial orbicularis palpebral heads to the medial canthal tendon (MCT) and maxilla bone. The marginal preciliary and retrociliary slips are not shown, as they are very small. *In vivo*, the orbital and preseptal orbicularis are closer to the MCT.

Deep heads

Superficial heads

KEY

1   Posterior lacrimal crest on lacrimal bone
2   Lacrimal fossa
3   Anterior lacrimal crest on frontal process of maxilla
4   Inferior orbital rim

PS   Preseptal orbicularis
PTH   Pretarsal (Horner's) orbicularis
PT   Pretarsal orbicularis
MCT   Medial canthal tendon
MC   Medial commissure
O   Orbicularis orbital portion

(near the puncta). It encircles the canaliculi along its route (Figure 1.7).

Medial canthal tendon

The medial canthal tendon (MCT) is the fibrous extension of orbicularis forwards onto the flat part of the ascending frontal process of the maxilla, and inserts as far as the naso-maxillary suture. Horizontal fibrous extensions from the tarsi extend into it. The inferior border of the MCT is well defined whilst the superior border blends with the superior fascia from the preseptal orbicularis (Figure 1.8).

From the anterior lacrimal crest the medial lacrimal fascia extends into the lacrimal fossa as far as the posterior lacrimal crest. The MCT blends with the periosteum in the superior part of the lacrimal fossa. It is perforated by the canaliculi. A thin posterior sheet of fascia passes to the posterior lacrimal crest in front of Horner's muscle, adherent to the lacrimal fascia (Figure 1.9).

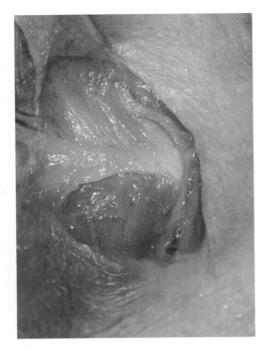

Figure 1.8

Dissection showing right medial canthal tendon. The preseptal orbicularis merges with the tendon and there is a free lower edge.

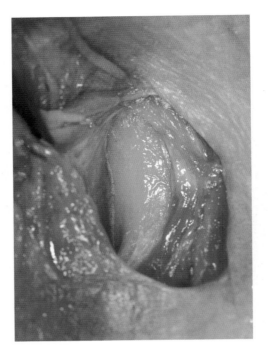

Figure 1.9

Medial canthal tendon, preseptal orbicularis and orbital periosteum reflected laterally to show the anterior lacrimal crest on the maxilla and view into the lacrimal fossa. The orbital periosteum and medial lacrimal fascia cover the lacrimal sac laterally.

Puncta and canaliculi

The puncta

These lie at the medial end of the upper and lower eyelids and open into the lacrimal lake adjacent to the junction of the plica semilunaris and bulbar conjunctiva. The upper punctum is normally between 0.5 and 1.0 mm more medial than the lower (in keeping with the plical curve), but when the eyelids are closed they are usually in contact. The puncta sit on top of a small elevation called the lacrimal papilla, are 0.2–0.3 mm in diameter and are surrounded by a ring of fibrous tissue. The lacrimal papillae are surrounded by pretarsal orbicularis fibres, which become deep heads at the posterior lacrimal crest and therefore pull the puncta medially and posteriorly. The medial ends of the lower lid retractors also help stabilize the puncta and prevent punctal eversion on blinking.

The canaliculi

The proximal canaliculi are short and vertical (approximately 2 mm), and then widen to form the ampulla before bending medially to form the horizontal part (8–10 mm long). The lower canaliculus is slightly longer than the upper, reflecting the more lateral position of the lower punctum. The canaliculi curve posteriorly and medially towards the lacrimal sac, in keeping with the normal medial eyelid curvature. They bend anteriorly after passing behind the MCT and meet at an angle of 25° to form the short common canaliculus (0–5 mm long).

The common canaliculus

Macrodacryocystography identifies the common caniculus (CC) in most adults (over 80 per cent) but it is less definable in infants. Common canalicular variations

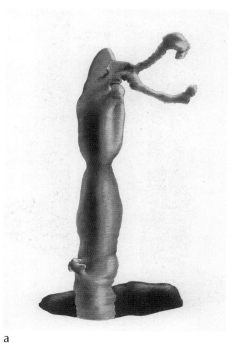

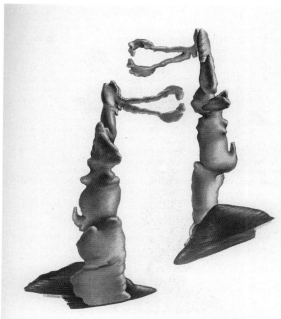

a

b

Figure 1.10

Original diagrams by Schaeffer (1912) of a right lacrimal system, based on histological serial sections.
a) Normal adult nasolacrimal passage, seen from behind and laterally.
b) Irregularity and diverticuli – lateral and medial view.
Schaeffer, J.P. (1912). Genesis of lacrimal passages in man. *Am. J. Anat.*, 13, 20–21, Figs 20-1. Copyright with permission from Wiley-Liss Inc., a subsidiary of John Wiley & Sons Inc.

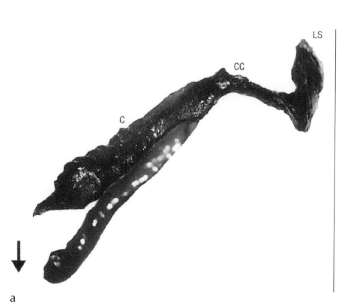

a

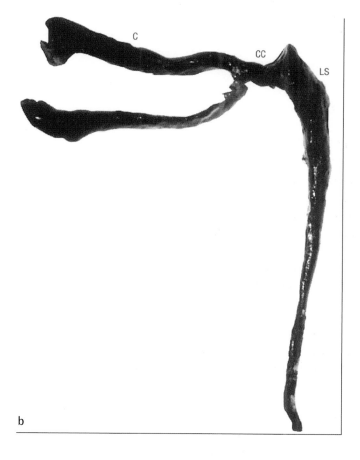

b

Figure 1.11

Rigid casts of the lacrimal drainage system by Tucker (1996).
a) Standard angle of entry (> 45°) of a left common canaliculus into the lacrimal sac. The cast is viewed from above.
b) Cast of a left lacrimal drainage system seen from the front.
Tucker, N.A. *et al.* (1996). The anatomy of the common canaliculus. *Arch. Ophthalmol.* Copyright, with permission American Medical Association.

a) STANDARD

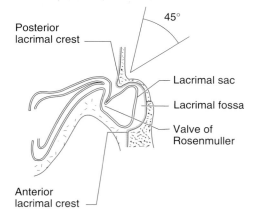

b) NON-REGURGITATING MUCOCOELE

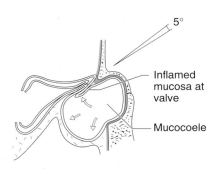

Figure 1.12

Diagram showing:
a)   Standard acute angle between common canaliculus and lacrimal sac
b)   How a mucocoele will reduce this angle, producing a potential one-way valve.

include separate openings into the sac, and a widening into the sac called the sinus of Maier. The CC is directed anteriorly before it enters the lacrimal sac, forming an acute angle with the sac (standard > 45°), as shown by Schaeffer in 1912 from reconstruction of histology sections (Figure 1.10).

Schaeffer's findings were confirmed by Tucker in 1996, from rigid methylmethacrylate casts of the canaliculi, sac and duct (Figure 1.11).

The initial antero-posterior direction of the canaliculi followed by the postero-anterior entry of the CC into the lacrimal sac is an important consideration when probing into the sac (see Chapter 3), and also explains non-regurgitating mucocoeles. The acute angle of entry of the CC into the sac creates a potential mucosal flap or valve across the opening – the valve of Rosenmuller. Distal or membranous CC obstruction caused by mucosal inflammation forms a partial canalicular obstruction, which can be overcome on syringing. The obstruction sometimes appears complete when a mucocoele expands the lacrimal sac anteriorly and medially, as this further reduces the angle of entry, compresses the canaliculus and closes the opening. There is a resultant one-way valve in which the sac is irrigated and inflated but no mucus is expressed. A similar 'one-way valve' is found in acute dacryocystitis and congenital dacryocoele (Figure 1.12).

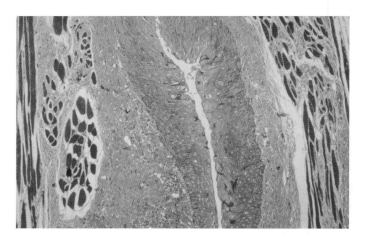

Figure 1.13

Histology of human lower canaliculus – longitudinal section. Note the surrounding orbicularis muscle fibres. With permission from Prof G. Ruskell.

Histology of the canaliculi

The ampulla and canaliculi are lined by non-keratinized stratified squamous epithelium. The histology of the lacrimal sac is very different from that of the canaliculi, with the transition occurring at the opening of the distal CC into the sac (Figure 1.13).

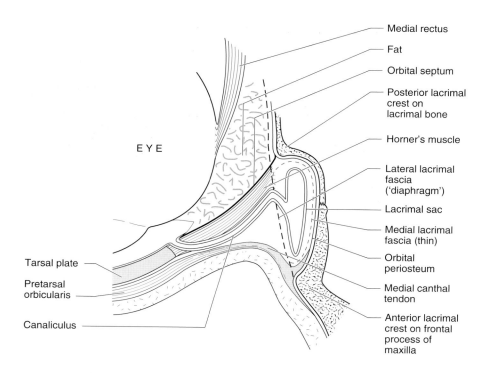

Medial rectus

Fat

Orbital septum

Posterior lacrimal crest on lacrimal bone

Horner's muscle

Lateral lacrimal fascia ('diaphragm')

Lacrimal sac

Medial lacrimal fascia (thin)

Orbital periosteum

Medial canthal tendon

Anterior lacrimal crest on frontal process of maxilla

EYE

Tarsal plate

Pretarsal orbicularis

Canaliculus

Figure 1.14

Cross-section of the lacrimal sac at the level of the medial canthal tendon.

Lacrimal sac

The sac is located in the lacrimal fossa on the anterior medial orbital wall. It lies entirely within the fossa unless expanded by a mucocoele or other swelling. Although it is within the bony orbit, it lies anterior to the orbital septum. The sac is 12–15 mm tall and 4–6 mm antero-posteriorly, but only 2–3 mm wide. The entrance of the common canaliculus is 3–5 mm below the apex of the sac – the sac above is called the fundus, and that below, the body. The widest part of the sac is a few millimetres from the apex. The sac wall is delicate, thin and often in apposition. The wall contains fibroelastic tissue arranged in a helical pattern, and the lumen is lined by non-keratinized stratified columnar epithelium.

The lacrimal fossa is lined by thin orbital periosteum, which is continuous with the periosteum over the frontal process of the maxilla and body of the maxilla. The periosteum is easily lifted off the bony fossa during external approach dacryocystorhinostomy. The lacrimal sac is enveloped on its supero-medial aspect by lacrimal fascia derived from the medial canthal tendon, which fuses with the periosteum. Thicker lacrimal fascia surrounds the sac laterally, between the anterior and

posterior lacrimal crests. The sac receives fibres from the deep heads of the pretarsal and preseptal orbicularis, the most important being Horner's muscle. This fascia has sometimes been called the lacrimal diaphragm because of the tear drainage function of Horner's muscle, which inserts into its upper part (Figure 1.14).

The orbital fat is located postero-laterally to the sac. Surgeons should be aware that during endonasal lacrimal surgery it is possible to enter the orbital fat accidentally, especially if the canaliculi are being kinked posteriorly by the light pipe. This risks causing orbital emphysema if the patient blows his or her nose, and should be avoided.

> **Surgical approaches to the lacrimal sac:**
> 1. External, through either a straight side of nose or a tear trough incision
> 2. Via the nose (transnasal or endonasal)
> 3. Transcanalicular.

Below the inferior edge of the MCT the sac is only covered by lacrimal fascia, orbicularis and skin. Since the normal sac lies flattened within the lacrimal fossa it does not really have an anterior surface, only an anterior border. An enlarged sac expands medially and anteriorly, and therefore it will have an anterior surface. Lacrimal sac fistulas track anteriorly through the soft lacrimal fascia and orbicularis to the skin surface. Dacryocystotomy (sac incision) for acute dacryocystitis is similarly through this soft tissue.

TIP

Lacrimal sac swellings are typically inferior to the anterior limb of the MCT, where the fascia is weak and can be stretched anteriorly. The tendon and fascia limit superior sac expansion.

TIP

Acute dacryocystitis does not spread posteriorly into the orbit to cause orbital cellulitis because the lacrimal sac is anterior to the orbital septum.

Blood supply of the lacrimal sac:
1. Branches of ophthalmic artery – dorsalis nasi, medial superior palpebral
2. External maxillary artery – angular branch of the facial artery
3. Internal maxillary artery – infra-orbital branch.

Venous drainage of the lacrimal sac:
A rich venous plexus surrounds the lacrimal sac as part of the substantia propria, but is much more prominent around the nasolacrimal duct. The veins drain to the angular vein.

Nerve supply of the lacrimal sac:
Infra-trochlear branch of the nasociliary nerve.

Histology of the lacrimal sac

The lacrimal sac is lined by non-keratinized stratified columnar epithelium with superficial goblet cells and a number of small mucus secretory glands and scattered foci of ciliated respiratory epithelium. There are serous glands in the fundus of the sac. The wall of the sac contains fibroelastic tissue in a helical pattern and some adenoid tissue. An inflamed mucocoele shows chronic inflammation of the stroma and increased mucus-producing goblet cells (Figure 1.15).

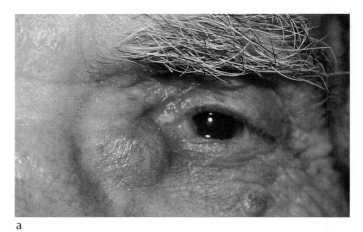

a

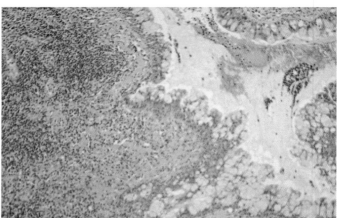

b

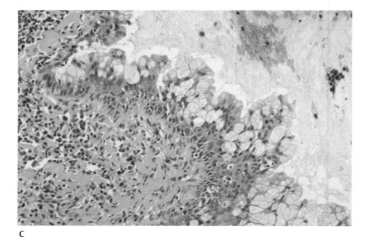

c

Figure 1.15
a) Left chronic mucocoele – intermittent dacryocystitis secondary to blocked nasolacrimal duct.
b) Histology of above lacrimal sac with chronic dacryocystitis showing chronic mucosal inflammation and extensive goblet cells with considerable intralumen debris. H&E ×100.
c) Higher power showing irregular epithelial surface with superficial fronds consisting mainly of goblet cells. H&E ×200.

Nasolacrimal duct

The proximal part of the nasolacrimal duct lies just within the lacrimal fossa. It is a continuation of the sac downwards to the inferior meatus and the nose. There is only a slight narrowing between a normal sac and nasolacrimal duct. The duct has an anterior–posterior orientation of approximately 15°; its route also slopes laterally from the top to the bottom with a slight convexity, in keeping with the slope of the lateral nasal wall.

> **TIP**
>
> *The sac and the duct appear anatomically continuous, but are separate structures. From the outside the difference lies in the more numerous and prominent veins surrounding the duct than the sac, and its thicker wall on incision. On the inside of the duct there is focal narrowing (valve of Krause).*

The nasolacrimal duct has an interosseous portion (approximately 12 mm) and an intermeatal portion (approximately 5 mm; see Figure 1.1). It opens into the nose on the anterior part of the lateral wall in the inferior meatus, approximately 10 mm posterior to the anterior end of the inferior turbinate and approximately 30 mm from the external nares (in an adult). The duct opening varies in size and shape, with a variable fold of mucosa, the valve of Hasner. The duct opens high up in the meatus or further down the lateral wall; sometimes a mucosal groove is seen below its opening in the inferior meatus.

> **TIP**
>
> *The nasolacrimal duct is close to the lateral nasal wall throughout its length and can be damaged during sino-nasal surgery (e.g. lateral rhinotomy for maxillary tumour) or functional endoscopic sinus surgery for sinus disease.*

> **TIP**
>
> *Diseases causing nasal mucosal inflammation can also involve the lower part of the nasolacrimal duct, resulting in its narrowing and eventual obstruction.*

The nasolacrimal duct is embedded in the bony nasolacrimal canal formed medially by a groove in the maxillary bone, and laterally by the lacrimal bone (above) and inferior turbinate bone (below). The lumen of the duct is narrow and its wall is thick in comparison with the lacrimal sac. Two-thirds of the canal is occupied by a venous plexus in the wall of the duct. This is surrounded by a continuation of the lacrimal fascia, which is adherent to the periosteum. The lumen of the duct may have diverticulae and areas of focal narrowing; these are either congenital valves (e.g. Krause) or as a result of inflammation rather than representing a completely healthy duct, and more information from intraduct micro-endoscopy is needed to clarify this.

> **Blood supply of the nasolacrimal duct:**
> 1. Ophthalmic artery – inferior palpebral branch of medial palpebral artery
> 2. Internal maxillary artery – infraorbital artery.

Histology of the nasolacrimal duct

The nasolacrimal duct is surrounded by a network of large capacitance vessels that connected to the 'cavernous' tissue of the inferior turbinate. The lamina propria contains the above venous plexus, loose connective tissue, a thin layer of elastic fibres, and many lymphocytic cells, sometimes arranged in follicles. The duct is lined with stratified columnar epithelium. The epithelial cells contain many vacuoles and lipid droplets, with

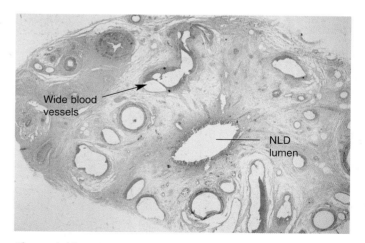

Figure 1.16

Histology cross-section of nasolacrimal duct showing thin lumen lined by stratified epithelium with a thick substantia propria containing wide capacitance blood vessels. With permission from Prof. G. Ruskell.

interspersed goblet cells. Ciliated respiratory epithelium, similar to nasal mucosa, is found near the valve of Hasner in the lower part of the duct (Figure 1.16).

Nose

The lacrimal surgeon requires a basic understanding of the sino-nasal anatomy.

The lower lacrimal system (sac and nasolacrimal duct) is in close proximity to the lateral nasal wall throughout its course, with tears draining into the inferior meatus and then posteriorly along the floor into the pharynx. Anterior ethmoid air cells extend close to the lacrimal fossa in most subjects. Lacrimal surgery involves entering the nose, whether doing a simple syringe and probing or dacryocystorhinostomy. Understanding the nasal anatomy is also important for pre-operative assessment and post-operative management of lacrimal patients, which often includes examining the nose.

The external nose

The nose protrudes from the mid-face. The soft tissues are supported by a skeleton consisting of the two nasal bones superiorly and the lateral cartilages inferiorly. The nasal septum forms most of the nasal bridge; it consists

of the vertical plate of the ethmoid bone, the vomer and several cartilages. The nostrils are separated by the columella. Nasal fractures may be associated with bony fractures around the nasolacrimal canal.

The nasal cavity

Most of the nose is inside the mid-face, with its axis at right angles to the facial plane. The nasal cavity or space is divided by the septum into two similar but asymmetrical parts. The initial entry area is the vestibule, lined by hair-bearing skin. The mucocutaneous junction lies beyond these hairs (vibrissae). Each nasal space has a floor, a narrow roof, a lateral nasal wall and medially the septum. Posteriorly, the nasal space enters the pharynx at the choana. The lacrimal surgeon should stay within the anterior third of the nose, anterior to the hiatus semilunaris and uncinate process on the lateral nasal wall.

The lateral nasal wall

This is the most important part of the nose for the lacrimal surgeon. It has important structures on it, which are seen as bumps, recesses and holes/openings – the latter from the paranasal sinuses and the nasolacrimal duct (Figure 1.17).

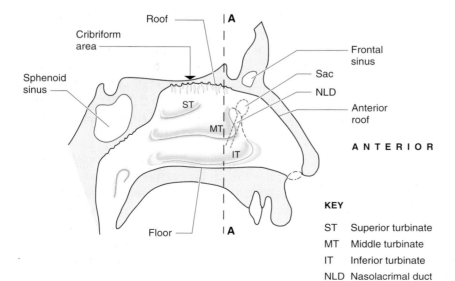

Figure 1.17

Diagram showing lateral nasal wall with position of underlying lacrimal sac and nasolacrimal duct. The endonasal lacrimal surgeon is advised to remain anterior to line AA in order to avoid the osteo-meatal complex (see Figure 1.23).

KEY

ST   Superior turbinate
MT   Middle turbinate
IT   Inferior turbinate
NLD Nasolacrimal duct

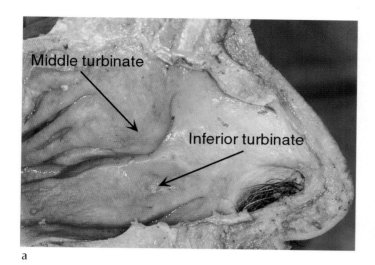
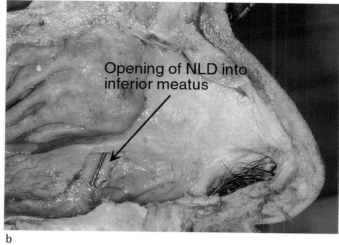

Figure 1.18

Dissections of a left lateral nasal wall showing a) the middle and inferior turbinates and b) a section of inferior turbinate removed to demonstrate a Bowman probe emerging from the nasolacrimal duct into the inferior meatus. NLD = nasolacrimal duct.

Structures on the lateral nasal wall:
1. Turbinates – inferior, middle, superior and, occasionally, supreme
2. Recesses – inferior meatus, middle meatus, superior meatus, hiatus semilunaris, frontal recess, spheno-ethmoidal recess
3. Air cells – agger nasi, bulla ethmoidalis
4. Other elevations – uncinate process
5. Holes/clefts/openings – nasolacrimal duct ostium, maxillary ostium, infundibulum, anterior and posterior ethmoid complex openings, frontal sinus ostium, sphenoidal ostium.

The inferior turbinate and meatus

The inferior turbinate is largest and occupies the lower third of the lateral nasal wall. Its anterior tip is located 1.5–2 cm inside the nasal space (adult). Its medial surface is usually concave and its lateral surface convex. The inferior turbinate is covered by thick vascular mucosa, which often makes it hypertrophied. Therefore examination of the nose is best done after applying a topical nasal decongestant, which shrinks the mucosa.

The nasolacrimal duct opening is on the lateral nasal wall in the inferior meatus, approximately 1 cm posterior to the anterior tip of the inferior turbinate. The opening is most commonly high up in the inferior meatus, and is visible with a 30° rigid Hopkins endoscope. It may have mucosal flap – the valve of Hasner. The shape of the opening varies considerably from round to slit-like, and to just a pit or fold with advanced nasolacrimal duct obstruction (Figure 1.18).

The middle turbinate and meatus

This turbinate is smaller and more elegant than the inferior turbinate. It is part of the ethmoid bone, and when enlarged by air cells is called a concha bullosa. These air cells usually originate from the agger nasi (see below). Other middle turbinate variations are described in Chapter 3. Normally its lateral wall is convex and its medial wall concave. It protects the middle meatus and its important physiological structures.

The anterior end of the middle turbinate is a constant anatomical landmark for lacrimal surgeons, since it relates closely to the position of the lacrimal sac. A swelling seen above the anterior end and superior to the middle turbinate is the agger nasi (Latin for nasal mound). It is a remnant of the first ethmoturbinal and is a pneumatized part of the lateral nasal wall, which can lie in the lacrimal fossa, between the lacrimal bone and

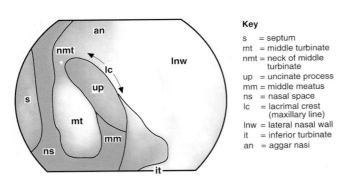

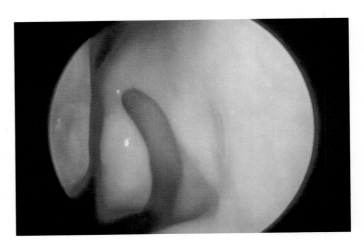

Figure 1.19

Diagram and nasal endoscopic appearance of a partially pneumatized middle turbinate, left lateral nasal wall.

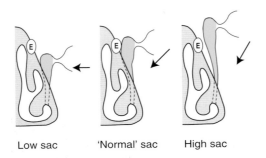

Figure 1.20

Diagrams showing the variation found between the lacrimal sac position and the structures on the lateral nasal wall. For simplicity, the size of the nasal space has been kept constant. If the sac is very high, it is inevitable that an ethmoid air cell will intervene between sac and nose.

the nasal space. The lacrimal crest, ridge or maxillary line is formed by the underlying frontal process of the maxilla and corresponds to the anterior surface of the nasolacrimal duct (Figure 1.19).

The relation of the lacrimal sac to the lateral nasal wall is variable; the sac may be relatively high, 'normal' or low compared to the adjacent anterior nasal space. This may simply reflect different sized nasal spaces and mid-face bony development. Anterior ethmoid air cells are found, to some extent, between the lacrimal fossa and

the lateral nasal wall in most subjects. These air cells are more common in the posterior superior lacrimal fossa. Recognizing these anatomical variations is important in dacryocystorhinostomy surgery (Figure 1.20).

The middle meatus contains the uncinate process, hiatus semilunaris (with the infundibulum) and ethmoid bulla. The uncinate process is seen as a smooth mucosal elevation in the anterior part of the middle meatus. *Uncinatus* is Latin for 'hook', and refers to the shape of a thin leaf of bone lying almost parallel to the lateral nasal wall. It is occasionally encountered in endonasal dacryocystorhinostomy if it extends anteriorly, partly overlying and in parallel to the lacrimal bone. However, usually the sac and duct lie immediately anteriorly and lateral to it and it does not need to be disturbed during surgery. It is a useful landmark in endonasal surgery. Its superior posterior free margin borders the hiatus semilunaris, which is an important crescent-shaped cleft leading to the infundibulum, into which the frontal, anterior ethmoid and maxillary sinuses drain (Figure 1.21).

The hiatus semilunaris is located between the uncinate process and the ethmoid bulla (Figure 1.22). The ethmoid bulla is a thin-walled bony prominence representing the largest and most consistent air cell of the anterior ethmoid complex, like a bleb on the lamina papyracea (medial wall of orbit).

The ethmoidal infundibulum is a funnel-shaped space bordered medially by the infundibulum and laterally by the lamina papyracea. The maxillary sinus ostium is

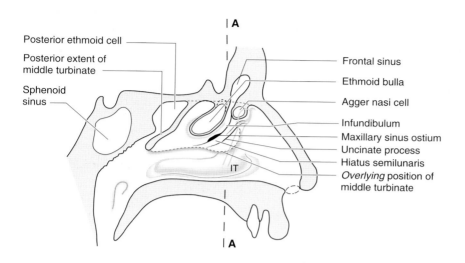

Posterior ethmoid cell
Posterior extent of middle turbinate
Sphenoid sinus

Frontal sinus
Ethmoid bulla
Agger nasi cell
Infundibulum
Maxillary sinus ostium
Uncinate process
Hiatus semilunaris
Overlying position of middle turbinate

IT

A

A

Figure 1.21

Diagram showing dissected left lateral nasal wall with middle turbinate removed to reveal the structures in the middle meatus, which include the uncinate process, hiatus semilunaris and infundibulum. These important structures to be avoided lie posterior to line AA.

KEY

IT Inferior turbinate

Yellow outline indicates *underlying* position of lacrimal sac and nasolacrimal duct.

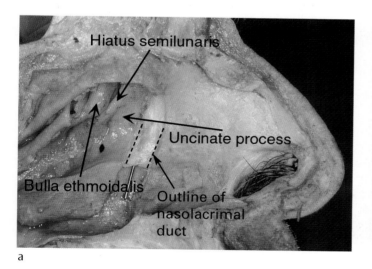

a

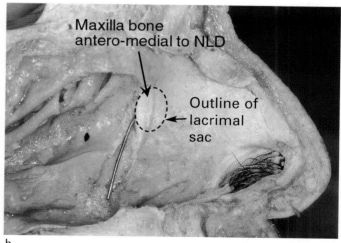

b

Figure 1.22

Dissection of left lateral nasal wall.
a)   The middle turbinate has been removed to show the proximity of the hiatus semilunaris. The mucoperiosteum overlying the nasolacrimal duct has been excised. Note that the uncinate is immediately posterior to the nasolacrimal duct.
b)   The remaining inferior turbinate bone and part of the lacrimal bone over the nasolacrimal duct (NLD) has been removed. The thick frontal process of the maxilla covers the antero-medial aspect of the upper NLD and lacrimal sac.

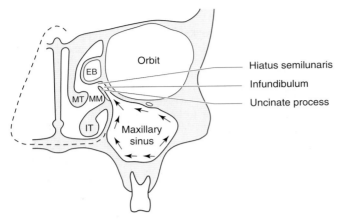

KEY

EB   Ethmoid bulla
MM   Middle meatus
MT   Middle turbinate
IT   Inferior turbinate

Figure 1.23

Diagram showing the hiatus semilunaris, infundibulum and uncinate process in the middle meatus – part of the osteo-meatal complex. The arrows show the normal maxillary mucociliary direction of flow and drainage.

found at the floor and lateral aspect of the infundibulum, where it is usually hidden from view by the fold of the uncinate process. The frontal sinus and anterior ethmoid complex drain into its superior part. The maxillary sinus drains via the posterior inferior part of the infundibulum into the middle meatus. This area is important pathophysiologically, as it forms part of the osteomeatal complex (see Physiology) (Figures 1.23, 1.24).

Practice point: The lacrimal surgeon will be able to recognize the main middle meatal structures and avoid them during surgery.

Details of the posterior part of the lateral nasal wall are less important to the lacrimal surgeon; the posterior ethmoid complex and sphenoid sinus drain into it.

Blood supply of the lateral nasal wall:
1.   External carotid origin – spheno-palatine branch of maxillary artery
2.   Internal carotid origin – anterior and posterior ethmoid arteries.

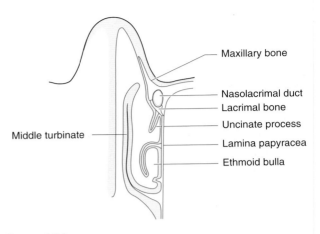

Figure 1.24

Diagram (sagittal section) showing position of the uncinate process in relation to the lacrimal bone and sac. There are several uncinate process anatomical variations e.g. medially rotated, where it is more prominent.

Venous drainage of the lateral nasal wall:
1.   Anterior part drains to the facial veins
2.   Roof drains to the ethmoid veins and into the ophthalmic vein.

The sphenopalatine artery enters the nose at the posterior end of the middle turbinate. It supplies the inferior and middle turbinates, i.e. inferior, middle and posterior part. The anterior and ethmoid arteries enter the nose at the junction of the roof and lateral wall. They supply the superior and anterior part. The blood vessels on the lateral nasal wall are highly anastomotic.

Nerve supply:
1.   Sensory supply – spheno-palatine, anterior and posterior ethmoid nerves
2.   Sympathetic supply – deep petrosal nerve to spheno-palatine ganglion
3.   Special sense of smell – olfactory nerves.

II. Osteology

1.   Skull bones
2.   Lacrimal fossa – constituents, relations and variations

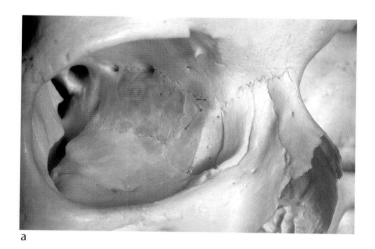

a

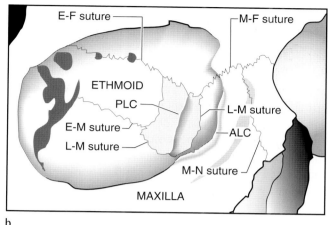

b

Figure 1.25

Right orbit.
a) Close-up view of right lacrimal fossa with equal amount of maxilla and lacrimal bone. Note the prominent indentation by the sutura notha (emissary vein) 2–3 mm anterior to the anterior lacrimal crest, which could be mistaken for a bony suture.
b) Diagram of above. E–F = ethmoid-frontal, E–M = ethmoid-maxillary, L–M = lacrimal maxillary, PLC = posterior lacrimal crest, ALC = anterior lacrimal crest, M–F = maxillary-frontal, M–N = maxillary-nasal.

3. Anterior air cells
4. Nasolacrimal canal – constituents, relations and variations
5. Maxillary bone
6. Lacrimal bone
7. Ethmoid bone.

Skull bones

Four skull bones are associated with the lacrimal drainage system:
1. Facial bone – maxilla
2. Lacrimal
3. Inferior turbinate
4. Cranial bone – ethmoid (including uncinate process).

TIP

Fracture of the middle turbinate during endonasal lacrimal surgery carries a risk of CSF leak by fracture of the cribriform plate, part of the ethmoid bone.

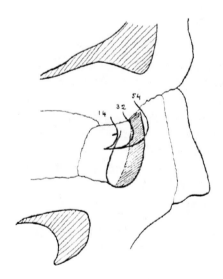

Figure 1.26

Original drawing by Whitnall (1911) showing how often the anterior ethmoid air cells were found in the upper lacrimal fossa when he examined 100 human skulls. With permission from the Royal Society of Medicine.

There are two bony lacrimal regions:
1. Orbital – lacrimal fossa
2. Nasal
   - nasolacrimal canal
   - inferior meatal.

Lacrimal fossa

The fossa is bordered anteriorly by the anterior lacrimal crest on the frontal (ascending) process of the maxilla and posteriorly by the posterior lacrimal crest on the lacrimal bone. The fossa shallows superiorly and ends by the lacrimal-frontal and maxillo-frontal sutures. Inferiorly the fossa becomes completely encircled by bone, when it becomes the nasolacrimal canal. The two bones forming the fossa (maxilla and lacrimal bone) join at the vertical lacrimal-maxillary suture within the fossa.

The fossa measures up to 8 mm antero-posteriorly, 16 mm vertically and 2–4 mm deep. Its vertical axis is slightly posterior, inferior and lateral.

The shape of the fossa varies – the anterior and posterior crests may be comparatively flat and the fossa shallow, or the crests prominent and the fossa deep. Either the maxilla or lacrimal bone may predominate; if the lacrimal bone predominates the floor is very fragile and easily removed during lacrimal surgery, if the maxilla predominates the floor is very dense (Figure 1.25; see also Figure 1.29).

Anterior air cells

In 1911, Whitnall demonstrated that ethmoid air cells are located medially to the upper part of the fossa (between the fossa and the nasal space) in approximately 90 per cent of skulls. In over 50 per cent of skulls, an agger nasi air cell extends into the frontal process of the maxilla as far as the anterior lacrimal crest. More recent computer tomographic evaluation of the normal ethmoid anatomy by Blaylock *et al.* in 1990 supports these original observations. Ethmoid air cells are entered in most patients when making the rhinostomy at dacryocystorhinostomy (Figure 1.26).

TIP
The ethmoid mucosa is thin and grey compared to pinker and thicker nasal mucosa.

Practice point: Recognize the anterior ethmoid air cells in the upper part of the lacrimal fossa during dacryo-cystorhinostomy and keep anterior and inferior to them, or go diagonally across, excising them, to reach the nasal space. A large agger nasi air cell can intervene between the lacrimal fossa and nasal space, in which case the rhinostomy must traverse its medial wall into the nose.

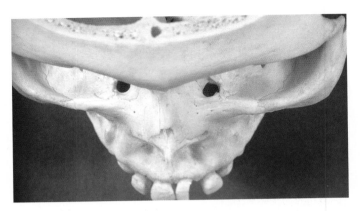

Figure 1.27

Bird's eye view of bony nasolacrimal canal openings in the anterior medial orbital floor.

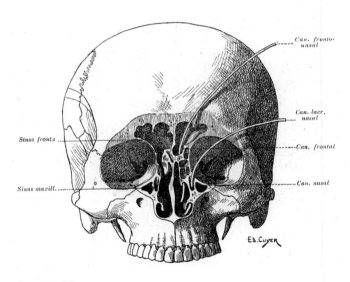

Figure 1.28

Original drawing by Poirier (1896) showing the upper probe from the frontal sinus into the middle meatus. The lower probe is in the nasolacrimal duct, showing its opening into the inferior meatus.

The nasolacrimal canal

The bony canal starts as a near-spherical opening in the infero-anterior orbital floor, approximately 3–5 mm from the rim. It becomes slightly oval as it descends, with the longer dimension antero-posterior.

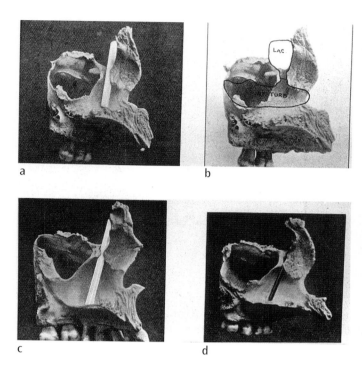

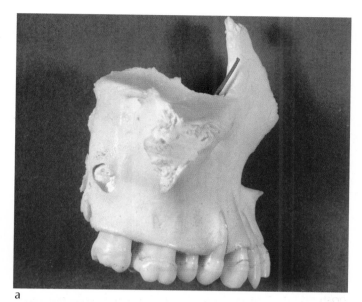

Figure. 1.29

Original photographs from Whitnall (1912) showing the variable maxilla contribution to the nasolacrimal canal (NLC).
a)   Standard maxilla contribution to NLC.
b)   Medial wall is formed by the lacrimal bone (LB) above and inferior turbinate (IT) below.
c)   and d) The upper part of the interosseous canal is increasingly maxilla-dominant and the canal correspondingly narrower.

With permission from the Royal Society of Medicine and the BMJ Publishing Group, copyright BMJ Publishing Group.

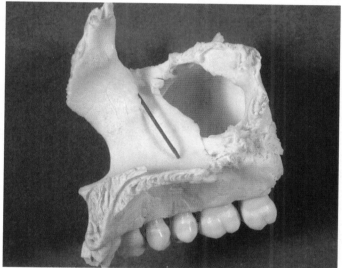

The interosseous part is approximately 12 mm long (see Figure 1.1) and inclines posteriorly (approximately 15°) and laterally, towards the first molar tooth. The lateral inclination relates to the size of the face – the narrower the interorbital distance and the wider the nose, the more lateral the course. The width of the bony canal is wider in men than women (Figures 1.27, 1.28).

Figure 1.30 *right*

Disarticulated right maxilla bone with green marker probe showing posterior lateral slope of nasolacrimal canal.
a)   Lateral aspect.
b)   Medial aspect. Canal sulcus on medial wall.
c)   Superior aspect. Maxilla bone partially encircling the opening.

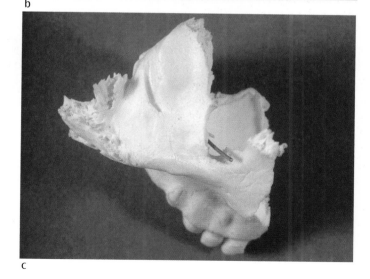

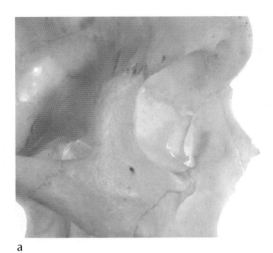

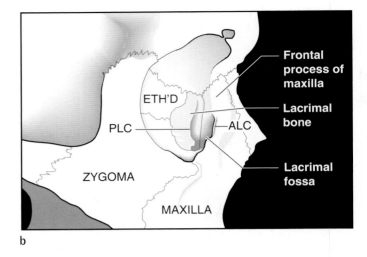

a   b

Figure 1.31

Right orbit.
a)   Lateral view of right lacrimal fossa. Transillumination shows the thin anterior part of lacrimal bone with a prominent
     posterior lacrimal crest and hamular process. Note the maxilla bone anterior to the lacrimal-maxillary suture is thick and
     transilluminates poorly.
b)   Diagram of above. PLC = posterior lacrimal crest, ALC = anterior lacrimal crest.

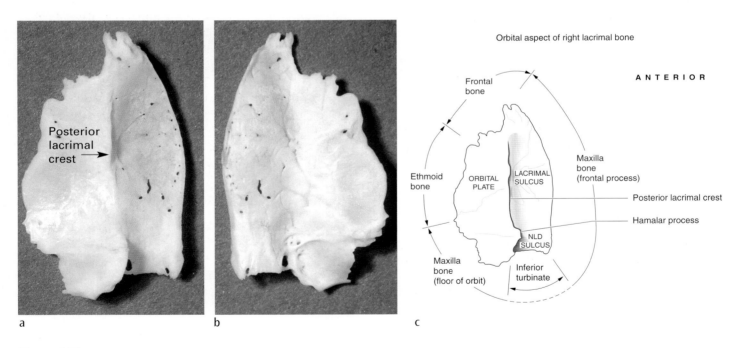

a   b   c

Figure 1.32

Disarticulated right lacrimal bone from a shallow lacrimal fossa. The posterior lacrimal crest has a faint process hamalaris at its
inferior end. Note the partially aerated and thin anterior lacrimal sulcus bone that forms the posterior lacrimal fossa.
a)   Orbital view.
b)   Nasal view.
c)   Diagram of lacrimal bone (orbital view) showing the bones that are articulating with it.

Comment: Groessl noted that the bony canal dimensions are smaller in women compared to men. He postulated that a narrower bony canal may partly explain the higher incidence of nasolacrimal duct obstruction in women.

Maxillary bone

The maxilla partly encircles the opening of the canal (anteriorly, laterally and posteriorly). In the interosseous portion, the lateral two-thirds of the canal are formed by the medial wall of the maxilla. The medial aspect is formed by the descending portion of the lacrimal bone in its upper part and the ascending part of the inferior turbinate bone below.

The proportion of lacrimal to maxilla bone on the medial aspect of the canal varies from mainly thin lacrimal bone to mainly thick maxilla (Figures 1.29, 1.30).

- Lacrimal bone dominant nasolacrimal canal.
- Maxilla bone dominant nasolacrimal canal.

Lacrimal bone

This fine bone is called the ossa unguis, as its size, shape and thin profile resembles a large toenail. It has an orbital aspect and a nasal aspect, with superior, inferior, medial and lateral sides. The orbital aspect forms part of the anterior medial orbital wall and lacrimal fossa. The posterior half (posterior to the posterior lacrimal crest) is thicker than the anterior half, which forms part of the lacrimal fossa. The process hamalaris (bony hook) at the lower end of the posterior lacrimal crest contributes in part to the opening of the nasolacrimal canal and articulates with the maxilla, which forms at least two-thirds of the opening (Figures 1.31, 1.32).

Ethmoid bone

The ethmoid bone occupies most of the space between the two orbits and forms part of the lateral wall of the nose, the roof and the central support. It includes the horizontal cribriform plates, and a midline vertical plate

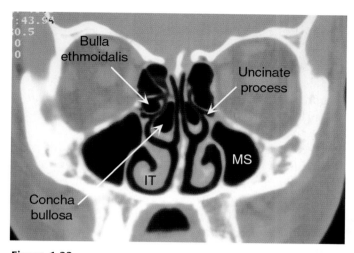

Figure 1.33

Coronal CT scan showing concha bullosa of middle turbinate (from a patient with thyroid eye disease, hence rectus muscles appear enlarged).

(crista galli and perpendicular plate) with lateral air cells. The thin lateral wall of the air cells forms part of the medial orbital wall (lamina papyracea), and the medial wall of the air cells forms the middle and superior turbinates. A pneumatized middle turbinate is called a concha bullosa. The ethmoid includes the agger nasi and ethmoid bulla, which are seen as mucosa-covered bulges on the lateral nasal wall. Occasionally, infra-orbital ethmoid air cells (Haller cells) lie in the orbital floor between the orbit and the maxillary sinus. The superior turbinate, if present, is part of the ethmoid bone (Figure 1.33).

Part B: Physiology of the lacrimal system

This is described under six headings:
1. Tear secretion
2. The lacrimal pump and tear drainage
3. Nasolacrimal duct functions – tear reabsorption
4. Rhinosinus physiology
5. Ageing changes
6. Tear drainage after dacryocystorhinostomy and Jones' tubes.

Tear secretion

The tear film is approximately 40 μm thick. This thickness decreases when the eyes are open, due to evaporation. The volume decreases with age and when the cornea is anaesthetized. The anterior lipid layer (adjacent to the air) is about 0.1 μm thick and is secreted mainly from the meibomian glands, with a bit coming from the glands of Zeis and Moll. The aqueous layer is about 7 μm thick, i.e. about 20 per cent of the total thickness. Aqueous tears are secreted by the lacrimal gland and the accessory glands of Krause and Wolfring. The mucin layer (adjacent to the cornea) is about 30 μm thick.

The conjunctival goblet cells produce the mucin that helps tear adhesion to the corneal epiphethial microvilli. Evaporation is reduced by superficial lipid and by eyelid closure.

The basal tear secretion rate equals the rate of tear drainage, evaporation and reabsorption. Increased tear production or decreased drainage results in a watering eye. The causes of hypersecretion and epiphora are covered in Chapter 2. Basal tear secretion is approximately 1.2 μl/min per day, total volume 10 ml per day. Reflex aqueous tear secretion, particularly from the lacrimal gland, increases this considerably (up to 100-fold). The conjunctival fornices hold 3–4 μl, the marginal tear strip 2–3 μl and the pre-corneal tear film 1 μl (Mishima, 1965).

The lacrimal pump and tear drainage

Adequate tear drainage depends on a functioning lacrimal pump mechanism initiated by the normal eyelid blink cycle. Tears enter the puncta at approximately 0.6 μl/minute (Maurice, 1973).

Tear meniscus to sac

Passive drainage

From the lacrimal lake there is a continual low rate of tear drainage into both puncta when the eyelids are not blinking, due to Krehbiel's phenomenon, capillary action and the normal eyelid downhill slope. There is some passive reflux back into the lacrimal lake.

Active drainage

Eyelid blinking distributes the pre-corneal tear film and propels the marginal tear strips medially towards the lacrimal lake and the puncta.

With blinking, the open puncta move towards each other and then occlude as they touch the lid margin. This squeezes the tears already in the ampulla into the

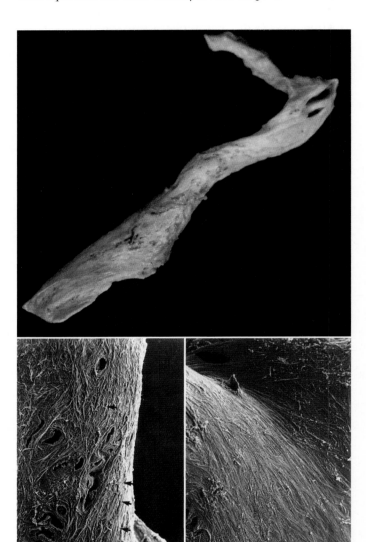

Figure 1.34

Top: isolated lacrimal system (canaliculi, sac and nasolacrimal duct) showing spiral appearance of outer collagen fibres. Lower pictures show scanning electron micrographs of spiral-arranged collagen and elastin fibres from duct. With kind permission of Andreas Thale (Thale *et al.*, 1998) and Springer–Verlag.

canaliculi. A Venturi effect may exist in the distal canaliculi, accelerating tear flow towards the common canaliculus and sac. Orbicularis contraction, including Horner's muscle (deep head pretarsal orbicularis), moves the eyelid medially. The canaliculi shorten and their lumen compress, thus increasing their intraluminal pressure and propelling the tears into the lacrimal sac (negative pressure). The lacrimal fascia is pulled laterally, which enables sac filling. A Bernoulli effect (suction) occurs in the ampulla and in the lacrimal sac. Once tears are in the sac, back-flow is reduced by the valve of Rosenmuller.

On eyelid opening with relaxation of Horner's muscle the tears enter the puncta secondary to reduced intra-canalicular pressure, completing the eyelid blink and the tear drainage cycle.

Lacrimal sac to nose

Passive drainage

Gravity and a suction effect assist sac emptying and flow down the nasolacrimal duct.

Active drainage

Contraction of Horner's muscle dilates the upper part of the lacrimal sac. It is believed that it also induces a peristaltic effect by compressing the lower sac, which helps drain tears out of the sac down the nasolacrimal duct. The peristaltic action caused by Horner's muscle contraction 'wrings out' the sac and duct in a cranial–caudal direction by the helical arrangement of the collagen and elastic fibres surrounding the naso-lacrimal duct, according to Thale (1998; Figure 1.34).

Nasolacrimal duct function – tear reabsorption

The tear flow rate from the lower end of the nasolacrimal duct is 10 times less than the tear flow entering the puncta. Reabsorption of tears occurs in the epithelium of the nasolacrimal duct. The large capacitance venous plexus then absorbs the fluid. Emptying of the venous plexus is facilitated by the 'wringing out' action described above (Thale, 1998).

Rhinosinus physiology

The paranasal sinuses and nose are lined by respiratory mucosa (ciliated columnar) with goblet cells. Mucociliary transport occurs in a particular pattern within the sinuses, beating towards the natural ostia. The anterior paranasal sinus complex (frontal sinus, agger nasi cells, anterior ethmoid and maxillary sinuses) drain via the ethmoidal infundibulum into the nasal cavity via the hiatus semilunaris. All these secretions empty into the middle meatus, and are then carried away by mucociliary transport towards the nasopharynx.

The osteo-meatal complex consists of:
- Lamina papyracea
- Uncinate process
- Bulla ethmoidalis
- Middle turbinate, middle meatus with the infundibulum and hiatus semilunaris (see Figures 1.23, 1.24).

The term 'osteo-meatal complex' refers to a functional anatomical unit. Anatomical variants, pathology and trauma can cause sinusitis from stenosis or obstruction of mucociliary drainage via the ethmoidal infundibulum.

History of functional endoscopic sinus surgery

Stammberger (1986) showed the importance of maintaining healthy nasal and sinus mucosa by his nasal endoscopic observations. This led to the development of functional endoscopic sinus surgery (FESS), where minimal, focal surgery within the nose and sinuses is performed under endoscopic visualization. This in turn led to endoscopic endonasal dacryocystorhinostomy.

Ageing changes

1. Reduction in tear quantity and quality after 40 years of age.
2. Lacrimal pump dysfunction
   - Increasing horizontal eyelid laxity and orbicularis descent

  ● Punctal eversion
  ● Eyelid malposition – entropion and ectropion.
3. Nasolacrimal duct stenosis
  ● Common in elderly. Women : men, 4 : 1.
Primary acquired nasolacrimal duct obstruction.
Gradual narrowing of the nasolacrimal duct lumen.
This is the result of a combination of swollen
mucosa and progressive fibrosis secondary to
chronic inflammation.

Tear drainage after dacrocystorhinostomy and Jones' tubes

Dacryocystorhinostomy

The tears emerge from the surgical ostium at the upper
end of the nasolacrimal duct/lacrimal sac, close to the
neck of the middle turbinate. Blinking assists drainage –
Horner's muscle pulls the lacrimal diaphragm laterally
and pumps the tears from the canaliculi into the 'sac'
area and then down the lateral nasal wall. This is clearly
visible when fluorescein instilled into the conjunctival
fornix is rapidly seen, by nasal endoscopy, at the ostium
(Figure 1.35).

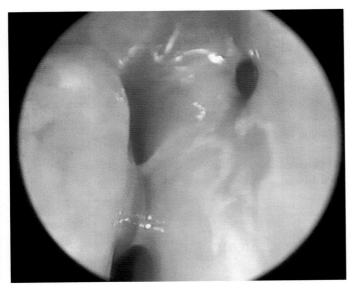

Figure 1.35
Endoscopic endonasal view of left functioning DCR ostium.
Fluorescein tears are seen trickling down the lateral nasal
wall. This is a positive functional endoscopic dye test (FEDT).

Jones' tubes

Tears pass down the glass bypass tube by capillary action
and gravity. The lacrimal pump function results in the
tube position rocking, which indirectly assists drainage.

Bibliography

Anatomy

Soft tissues:

Bailey, J. H. (1923). Surgical anatomy of the lacrimal sac. *Am.
J. Ophthalmol.*, 6, 665–71.

Calhoun, K. H., Rotzer, W. H. and Stiernberg, C. M. (1990).
Surgical anatomy of the lateral nasal wall. *Otolaryngol. Head
Neck Surg.*, 1032, 156–60.

Horner, W. E. (1823). Description of a small muscle at the
internal commissure of the eyelids. *J. Med. Phys.*, 8, 70–80.

Jones, L. T. (1961). An anatomical approach to problems of
the eyelids and lacrimal apparatus. *Arch. Ophthalmol.*, 66,
137–50.

Patton, J. M. (1923). Regional anatomy of the tear sac. *Ann.
Otol. Rhinol. Laryngol.*, 32, 58–60.

Royer, J., Adenis, J. P., Bernard, J. A. *et al.* (1982). *L'appareil
Lacrymal*, pp. 165–250. Masson.

Schaeffer, J. P. (1912). The genesis and development of the
nasolacrimal passages in man. *Am. J. Anat.*, 13, 1–24.

Tucker, N. A., Tucker, S. M. and Linberg, J. V. (1996). The
anatomy of the common canaliculus. *Arch. Ophthalmol.*, 114,
1231–4.

Osteology:

Blaylock, W. K., Moore, C. A. and Linberg, J. V. (1990).
Anterior ethmoid anatomy facilitates dacryocystorhinostomy.
Arch. Ophthalmol., 108, 1774–7.

Groessl, S. A., Sires, B. S. and Lemke, B. N. (1997). An
anatomical basis for primary acquired nasolacrimal duct
obstruction. *Arch. Ophthalmol.*, 115, 71–4.

Hartikainen, J., Aho, H. J., Seppa, H. *et al.* (1996). Lacrimal
bone thickness at the lacrimal sac fossa. *Ophthalmic Surg.
Lasers*, 27, 679–84.

Patton, J. M. (1923). Regional anatomy of the tear sac. *Ann.
Otol. Rhinol. Laryngol.*, 32, 58–60.

Poirier, P. (1896). *Traite d'anatomie Humaine*. Masson.

Whitnall, S. E. (1911). The relations of the lacrimal fossa to
the ethmoid air cells. *Ophthal. Rev.*, 30, 321–5.

Whitnall, S. E. (1912). The nasolacrimal canal: the extent to which it is formed by the maxilla and the influence of this upon its calibre. *Ophthalmoscope*, 10, 557–8.

Tear drainage:

Becker, B. B. (1992). Tricompartmental model of the lacrimal pump mechanism. *Ophthalmology*, 99, 1139–45.

Doane, M. G. (1981). Blinking and the mechanics of the lacrimal drainage system. *Ophthalmology*, 88, 844–50.

Jones, L. T. (1957). Epiphora II. Its relation to the anatomic structure and surgery of the medial canthal region. *Am. J. Ophthalmol.*, 43, 203–12.

Maurice, D. M. (1973). The dynamic drainage of tears. *Int. Ophthalmol. Clin.*, 13, 103–116.

Mishima, S., Gasset, A., Klyce, S. and Baum, J. (1966). Determination of tear volume and tear flow. *Invest. Ophthalmol.*, 5, 264–76.

Rosengren, B. (1972) On lacrimal drainage. *Ophthalmologica*, 164, 409–21.

Thale, A., Paulsen, F., Rochels, R. and Tillmann, B. (1998). Functional anatomy of the human efferent tear ducts: a new theory of tear outflow mechanism. *Graefe's Arch. Clin. Exp. Ophthalmol.*, 236, 674–8.

Sinus surgery:

Stammberger, H. (1986). Endoscopic endonasal surgery – concepts in treatment of recurrent rhinosinusitis. Part 1. Anatomic and pathophysiologic considerations. *Otolaryngol. Head Neck Surg.*, 94, 143–7.

CHAPTER 2

Causes of a Watering Eye

The causes of a watering eye are:

1. Hypersecretion
2. Epiphora
3. Combined hypersecretion and epiphora.

It is essential to distinguish between these and to recognize that hypersecretion and epiphora may coexist.

Definitions

Hypersecretion

Hypersecretion is an excessive production of tears. It is also referred to as lacrimation, hyperlacrimation and reflex tearing.

Epiphora

Epiphora is a result of reduced tear outflow, i.e. defective tear drainage. Exclude causes of hypersecretion.

An accurate history and systematic examination of the eyelids, ocular surface and lacrimal system enables the examiner to distinguish between hypersecretion and epiphora. This is important, as the treatment of hypersecretion is largely medical, and that of epiphora surgical.

Combined hypersecretion and epiphora

Some eyelid and external eye conditions result in both lacrimation and epiphora:
1. Lower lid ectropion with inflamed keratinized exposed tarsal conjunctiva
2. Hay fever causes hypersecretion and epiphora when the conjunctiva, lacrimal sac, nasolacrimal duct and nasal mucosa are oedematous
3. Involutional lower lid entropion causes hypersecretion by the irritant effect of the inturning lid and lashes, and epiphora because the lower punctum is not in the correct position to drain the tears and the overriding orbicularis is an ineffective lacrimal pump
4. Patients with thyroid eye disease have hypersecretion from exposure keratitis and mild epiphora from defective orbicularis action (stretched) and canalicular function (compressed) from proptosis
5. Patients with facial palsy have hypersecretion from lagophthalmos and exposure keratitis, as well as epiphora from lacrimal pump dysfunction.

Absence of epiphora with blocked nasolacrimal duct

Tear production and drainage are normally in balance.

> Practice point: Symptoms of epiphora only occur when outflow resistance exceeds tear production.
> Some elderly patients with, for example, a complete nasolacrimal duct block do not complain of epiphora since they also have an age-related reduction in tear production.

Causes of hypersecretion

Two common causes of hypersecretion are staphyloccocal lid margin disease (blepharitis) and ocular surface disease (dry eye). Paradoxical symptoms of watering occurring with blepharitis, and dry eyes are usually bilateral, worse in a dry smoky atmosphere and at the end of the day. Hypersecretion is chronic.

Causes of unilateral lacrimation include corneal abrasion, corneal foreign body and keratitis, for example marginal keratitis or viral keratitis. These cause acute lacrimation from trigeminal sensory nerve irritation (Figure 2.1).

External eye examination

Exclude the common causes of hypersecretion by clinical examination of the external eye on the slit-lamp, with and without guttae fluorescein and Rose Bengal. Measure the tear break-up time and do a Schirmer's test.

NB: If Rose Bengal is used, wash out afterwards with saline because it stings considerably after the topical anaesthetic wears off.

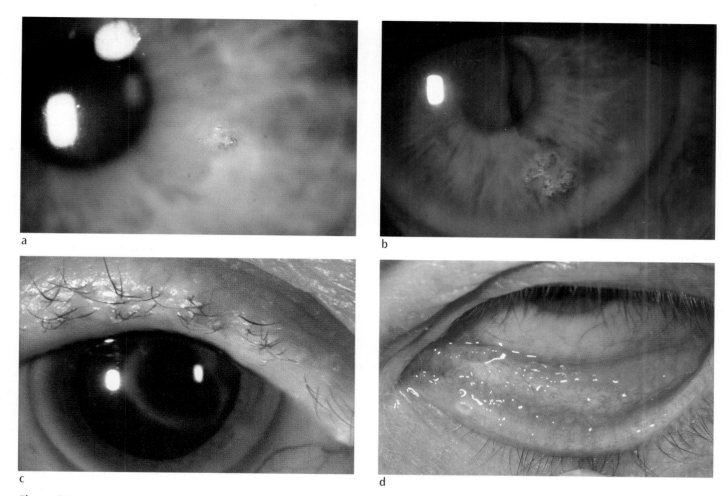

Figure 2.1

Examples of causes of hyperlacrimation:
a) Corneal rust ring
b) Herpes simplex keratitis
c) Anterior blepharitis with eyelash collarettes
d) Follicular conjunctivitis from molluscum contagiosum.

Blepharitis

Examine the anterior and posterior lid margins.

Anterior lid margin disease is indicated by lash root collarettes and debris, with a telangiectatic anterior lid margin.

Posterior lid margin disease is indicated by posterior lid margin pitting with loss of normal architecture, posterior marginization of the meibomian openings (opening onto the tarsal conjunctival surface) and posterior lid margin telangiectasia.

Dry eyes

In dry eyes, the tear meniscus may be low or elevated (if there is reflex tearing). The tear film may contain debris – lipid, mucin, flakes and filaments. Use guttae fluorescein to stain areas of corneal and conjunctival epithelial defects, and Rose Bengal to show extensive mucin-deficient areas and filaments. Observe the tear break-up time with fluorescein (less than 10 seconds is abnormal). Do a Schirmer's test, but be aware that results can be unreliable as it induces reflex tearing, even with topical anaesthesia, due to lid margin irritation.

Consider a trial of lid hygiene and topical lubricants if indicated.

If in doubt, refer the patient to an external eye disease specialist for an opinion.

Causes of hypersecretion:
1. Supranuclear (CNS) – emotion and voluntary crying.
2. Reflex tearing – trigeminal nerve stimulation. Lid margin disease (e.g. blepharitis and trichiasis). Conjunctival disease (e.g. vernal catarrh and hay fever conjunctivitis). Corneal disease (e.g. dry eye, corneal foreign body, keratitis, contact lens related problem). Ocular inflammation (e.g. iritis).
3. Other – bright lights, yawning, sneezing.
4. Infranuclear – facial nerve aberrant innervation/regeneration, crocodile tears.
5. Lacrimal gland stimulation – dacryoadenitis and pharmacological, e.g. cholinergic agents.

Causes of epiphora

There are congenital and acquired causes of epiphora. The most common cause in the first 2 years of life is congenital nasolacrimal duct obstruction. In adults, especially the elderly, the most common causes are acquired nasolacrimal duct stenosis, lower eyelid malposition, or both. A complete obstruction of the nasolacrimal duct is fairly easy to diagnose, whereas partial nasolacrimal duct stenosis causing functional epiphora is more difficult to confirm.

Obstruction at any point along the lacrimal drainage pathway, from the punctum to the nose, can cause epiphora. Symptoms range from tears overflowing onto the cheek in severe lacrimal drainage impairment, to intermittent epiphora with a partial block. Symptoms are unilateral or bilateral. Epiphora is typically worse in winter months and windy weather. The eye can be sticky due to an expressible mucocoele or collected dried tears. The vision can be blurred secondary to an elevated tear meniscus (prismatic effect – especially on down-gaze, for example when reading) or tear-splattered glasses. Chronic epiphora can cause red, sore lower-lid skin, with secondary anterior lamella (vertical) shortening (mild cicatricial ectropion). Excessive wiping away of tears can cause or exacerbate a medial ectropion.

Functional epiphora

Functional. 'Affecting the functions only, not structural.'
Functio: Latin for perform.
(From the *Shorter Oxford English Dictionary*.)

This term is used when there is epiphora with patent syringing, in the absence of any causes of hypersecretion.

The most common cause is narrowing or stenosis of the nasolacrimal duct, which increases the resistance to tear outflow but does not cause a complete anatomical obstruction, called functional nasolacrimal duct obstruction.

The term 'lacrimal pump dysfunction' is used for orbicularis causes of reduced tear drainage – e.g. of paralytic aetiology.

Common causes of functional epiphora:
1. Facial palsy with paralytic ectropion
2. Punctal stenosis
3. Single functioning canaliculus
4. Common canalicular stenosis
5. Narrowing or irregularity of the nasolacrimal duct causing physiological dysfunction of tear drainage.

Stenosis. 'The contraction or stricture of a passage, duct, or canal.'
Stenos: Greek for narrow.
(From the *Shorter Oxford English Dictionary*.)

Obstruction. 'The hindering or stopping of the course. Anything that stops or blocks a way or passage.'
Obstructio: Latin for block.
(From the *Shorter Oxford English Dictionary*.)

Classification of epiphora

There are many causes of epiphora. An anatomical classification helps develop a systematic approach to the examination and choice of surgery:

1. Lacrimal pump, eyelid, puncta and conjunctiva
2. Canaliculi, sac and nasolacrimal duct
3. Nose.

Lacrimal pump, eyelid, puncta and conjunctiva

Lacrimal pump problems causing epiphora

1. Horizontal lid laxity – floppy eyelid and lax eyelid syndromes and involutional ectropion and entropion (± mid-face ptosis and orbital fat protrusion)
2. Lower lid entropion with ineffective overriding orbicularis muscle
3. Lower lid ectropion with ineffective orbicularis muscle, e.g. paralytic, cicatricial – burn, scar, scleroderma, varix
4. Loss of skin/orbicularis – tissue replacement, e.g. after tumour excision.

Eyelid malposition causing epiphora

Lower lid ectropion:
1. Involutional:
   - Punctal medialization
   - Punctal eversion
   - Medial
   - Total eversion.
2. Mechanical:
   - Tumour (e.g. basal cell carcinoma, neurofibroma).
3. Cicatricial:
   - Actinic (sun-damaged)
   - Post-blepharoplasty
   - Traumatic contact dermatitis.

Lower lid entropion:
1. Involutional (in-turning lashes and skin–ocular contact also cause hypersecretion)
2. Cicatricial (trichiasis also causes hypersecretion).

Conjunctival causes of epiphora

1. Conjunctivochalasis – occludes punctum and may interfere with tear movement along the lower lid (lacrimal pump)
2. Allergic conjunctivitis.

Punctal causes of epiphora

1. Congenital agenesis or imperforate
2. Acquired occlusion or stenosis
   - Dry punctum from non-use in chronic ectropion
   - Post-infection
   - Post-irradiation
   - Pharmacological – e.g. topical antiviral (g Idoxuridine), anti-glaucoma (g Eppy and phospholine iodide), systemic (5-fluorouracil)
   - Conjunctival – ocular cicatricial pemphigoid and Stevens–Johnson Syndrome
   - Burns
   - Tumours – ampulla mucosal papilloma
   - Punctal occlusion for dry eye.
3. Malposition
   - Punctal medial displacement
   - Medial ectropion
   - Centurion Syndrome (anterior displacement of medial canthal tendon on maxilla).

Canaliculi, sac and nasolacrimal duct

Canalicular causes of epiphora (Figure 2.2)

1. Congenital absence or fistula
2. Acquired – intrinsic
   - Post-herpetic infection (simplex and varicella zoster)
   - Infective canaliculitis
   - Trauma, including surgical (pigtail probe, lacrimal surgery, tumour excision)
   - Post-irradiation
   - Pharmacological – as for puncta
   - Tumour.
3. Acquired – extrinsic
   - Compression/invasion and occlusion by adjacent tumour, e.g. basal cell carcinoma, squamous cell carcinoma, lymphoma, neurofibroma.

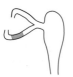
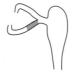

Focal mid lower   Focal distal lower   Extensive upper
                                             and lower

Figure 2.2

Diagram showing canalicular causes of epiphora.

Common canalicular (CC) causes of epiphora

- Distal CC (towards the sac) = membranous obstruction
- Proximal CC (towards the tear film) = fibrous obstruction.

Membranous obstruction occurs at the medial end – valve of Rosenmuller – at the junction of the common canaliculus and sac. This occurs secondary to mucosal inflammation. It may exist alone, or be associated with nasolacrimal duct stenosis. It is commonly a mild constriction felt as a 'pop' during probing. More severe block exists, which is difficult to overcome with probing without causing discomfort, especially if there is a non-expressible mucocoele.

Proximal obstruction is fibrous obstruction at the lateral end of the common canaliculus. It occurs most commonly after herpetic infection. (See also other causes of canalicular obstruction). It is unlikely to be overcome by probing (Figure 2.3).

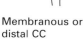

Membranous or   Fibrous or
distal CC   proximal CC

a   b

Figure 2.3

Diagram showing difference between distal (a) and proximal (b) common canalicular (CC) obstruction.

Lacrimal sac causes of epiphora

1. Diverticulum/outpouching of sac
2. Fistula from sac to nose or cheek
3. Trauma
4. Inflammation
   - Extension of primary acquired nasolacrimal duct obstruction (±dacryoliths)
   - Wegener's granulomatosis
   - Sarcoidosis
   - Allergy/hayfever
5. Tumour – extrinsic or intrinsic.

Lacrimal sac tumours

Extrinsic – compressing or invading the sac from the outside:
- Basal cell carcinoma
- Squamous cell carcinoma
- Lymphoma
- Neurofibroma
- Other.

Intrinsic – arising from the sac walls:
1. Epithelial
   - Papilloma (exophytic or endophytic)
   - Carcinoma (squamous, transitional cell, adenocarcinoma, mucoepidermoid)
   - Other
2. Non-epithelial
   - Lymphoma
   - Melanoma
   - Leukaemia
   - Metastases
   - Haemangioma
   - Neurofibroma
   - Other.

Nasolacrimal duct causes of epiphora (Figure 2.4)

1. Primary acquired nasolacrimal duct obstruction – commonest cause in adults
2. Secondary acquired lacrimal obstruction, including:

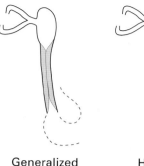
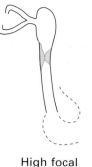
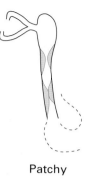
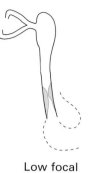

Generalized   High focal   Patchy   Low focal

Figure 2.4
Diagram of nasolacrimal duct stenosis/obstruction in adults, which can be patchy or generalized, partial or complete, high or low focal.

- Trauma – including lateral rhinotomy and FESS (functional endoscopic sinus surgery)
- Tumour – as for sac; especially extension from maxillary sinus
3. Congenital nasolacrimal duct obstruction
  - Delayed opening of valve of Hasner ± dacryocoele
  - Part of craniofacial abnormality
  - Nasolacrimal duct agenesis (rare).

Clinical findings of PANDO:

1. Epiphora
   - Partially blocked nasolacrimal duct = functional epiphora
   - Totally blocked nasolacrimal duct = epiphora
2. Mucocoele
3. Acute dacryocystitis – usually associated with a total block, but exceptions if partitioned sac or sac diverticulum
4. ± distal common canalicular obstruction
5. Dacryoliths = inspissated mucus and cellular debris.

Primary acquired nasolacrimal duct obstruction

Linberg coined the term 'primary acquired nasolacrimal duct obstruction' (PANDO) in 1986 to describe the most common cause of epiphora in adults. The pathogenesis of PANDO is believed to be chronic mucosal inflammation with progressive fibrosis and narrowing of the nasolacrimal duct within the rigid nasolacrimal canal. Inflammation can extend up into the lacrimal sac and affect the common opening (valve of Rosenmuller), resulting in coexistent membranous occlusion. Increased venous stasis within the venous sinusoids around the nasolacrimal duct may also play a role.

PANDO occurs in older people, affecting women more than men. It covers a spectrum of disease from slight narrowing to complete obstruction. Stenosis therefore precedes complete obstruction, during which time syringing is patent, often with regurgitation. The increasing outflow resistance causes functional epiphora prior to full obstructive epiphora.

Nose

Nasal causes of epiphora

1. Allergic rhinitis
2. Severe rhinosinus disease (polyps)
3. Iatrogenic – from previous nasal surgery – lateral rhinotomy or FESS
4. Tumours – spread to lacrimal sac and nasolacrimal duct from nasal space and/or adjacent sinuses (e.g. inverted papilloma and squamous cell carcinoma).

Nasal causes of epiphora are rare.

Table 2.1 Bartley's SALDO classification

Aetiology	Condition	Puncta	Canaliculi	Sac	NL duct
Infections	**Bacterial**				
	• Actinomycoses	+	+		
	• Chlamydia	+	+		
	Viral				
	• Herpes simplex	+	+		
	• Herpes zoster	+	+		
	Fungal				
	• Aspergillus	+	+	+	
	• Candida	+	+	+	
	Parasitic	+	+	+	+
Inflammations	**Endogenous**				
	• Wegener's			+	+
	• Sarcoidosis			+	+
	• Cicatricial pemphigoid	+	+		
	• Stevens–Johnson Syndrome	+	+		
	Exogenous				
	• Eyedrops	+	+		
	• Radiation	+	+		
	• Fluorouracil	+	+		
	• Allergy	+	+		
	• Burns	+			
	• 'Pyogenic granuloma'		+	+	+
Neoplasia	**Primary**				
	• Papilloma	+	+	+	
	• Squamous cell carcinoma		+	+	+
	• Lymphoma			+	
	• Haemangiopericytoma			+	
	Secondary				
	• Adenocystic carcinoma			+	
	• Basal cell carcinoma		+	+	
	• Leukaemia			+	
	• Lymphoma		+	+	
	• Squamous cell carcinoma		+	+	
	Metastatic				
	• Breast carcinoma			+	
	• Melanoma			+	
	• Prostatic carcinoma			+	
Trauma	**Medical therapy**				
	• Iatrogenic				
	• Punctal plugs	+	+		
	• Probing		+		
	• Silicone intubation		+		
	• Sinus surgery				+
	• Nasal surgery				+
	Accidental trauma				
	• Soft tissue laceration		+	+	
	• Bony duct fracture			+	+
Mechanical	**Internal**				
	• Dacryolith		+	+	+
	• Migrated or retained medical device (e.g. punctal plug)		+	+	+
	External				
	• 'Kissing puncta'	+			
	• Conjunctivochalasis	+			
	• Frontal/ethmoidal mucocoele			+	+

Secondary acquired lacrimal drainage obstruction

The term 'secondary acquired lacrimal drainage obstruction' (SALDO) was adopted in 1992 by Bartley to cover the wide range of secondary causes of epiphora from infections, inflammation, neoplasia, trauma and mechanical. Any part of the lacrimal drainage system could be affected, including the nasolacrimal duct. The causes have been largely covered in the anatomical classification of epiphora used above.

Bartley's SALDO classification is summarized in Table 2.1.

Bibliography

Bartley, G. B. (1992, 1993). Acquired lacrimal drainage obstruction: an aetiologic classification system, case reports, and a review of the literature. *Ophthal. Plastic Reconstr. Surg.*, 8, 237–249 and 9, 11–26.

Linberg, J. V. and McCormick, S. A. (1986). Primary acquired nasolacrimal duct obstruction: a clinicopathologic report and biopsy technique. *Ophthalmology*, 93, 1055–62.

Stefanyszyn, M. A., Hidayat, A. A., Pe'er, J. J. and Flanagan, J. C. (1994). Lacrimal sac tumours. *Ophthal. Plastic Reconstr. Surg.*, 10, 169–84.

CHAPTER 3

Lacrimal Assessment

In this chapter the techniques for examining a patient with epiphora are described. The causes of a watering eye and the importance of distinguishing between hypersecretion and epiphora have already been discussed in Chapter 2

Part A: Periorbital, lid and lacrimal system
Part B: Nasal examination
Part C: Radiology

History

An accurate history must be taken, incorporating the patient's symptoms, past ophthalmic, nasal and medical histories, and any allergies and drugs. Exclude causes of hyper- and hypo-secretion of tears by examining the lid margins, conjunctiva, tear film and cornea on the slit lamp. Then examine the lacrimal system systematically, using a standard approach.

Examination

The lacrimal examination consists of three parts:

A Periorbital, lid and lacrimal system assessment
- Observe the face, including the forehead and cheeks, the periorbital and medial canthal areas and the eyelids
- Do a slit-lamp examination of the puncta and external eye and measure the tear meniscus
- Perform dye tests
- Syringe the lacrimal system.

B Nasal examination
- Do an endonasal examination with a rigid telescope to exclude nasal causes of epiphora and identify the anatomical variations that influence the outcome of surgery.

C Radiology – do the following ancillary radiological investigations, as indicated.
- Macrodacryocystography
- Nuclear lacrimal scintigraphy
- Computer tomography or magnetic resonance imaging of the lacrimal system and sinuses.

The findings from this standard approach will differentiate epiphora from hypersecretion of tears, and locate the most likely site and cause of epiphora. No single test should be relied on without considering the findings of all the tests to build up an accurate picture.

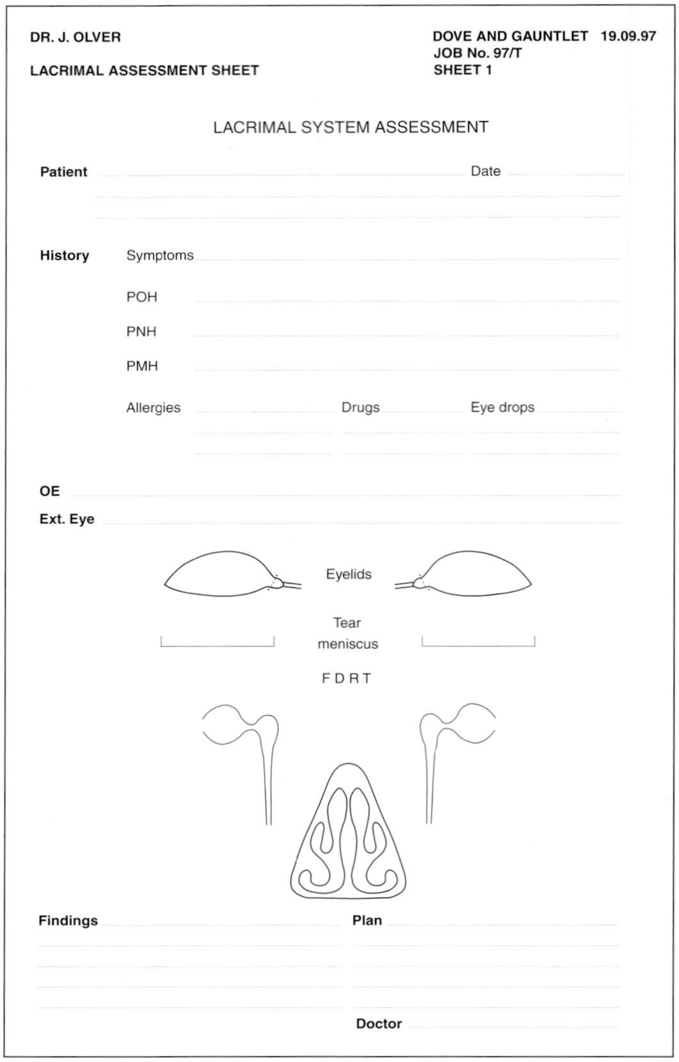
DR. J. OLVER
LACRIMAL ASSESSMENT SHEET
DOVE AND GAUNTLET 19.09.97
JOB No. 97/T
SHEET 1

LACRIMAL SYSTEM ASSESSMENT

Patient Date

History Symptoms
POH
PNH
PMH
Allergies Drugs Eye drops

OE
Ext. Eye

Findings Plan

Doctor

Figure 3.1

Lacrimal assessment proforma. Published with permission from *Eye*.

It is useful to have a prepared sheet on which to record the findings of the lacrimal assessment. A simple one is suggested (Figure 3.1). The use of diagrams helps to clarify the findings, both for the examiner and for easy interpretation by others.

Part A: Periorbital, lid and lacrimal system assessment

General examination of the face and periorbital region

Look for facial and periorbital asymmetry, lumps, bulges, mid-face ptosis and eyelid malposition. Simple observation combined with a careful history is the key to success in the lacrimal assessment. Look for the unexpected.

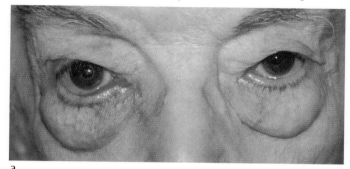

a

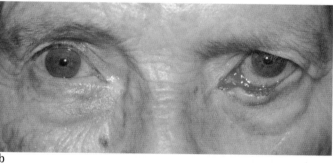

b

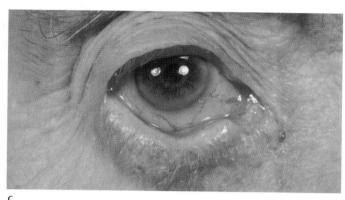

c

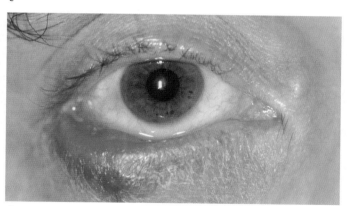

d

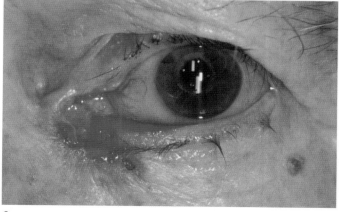

e

Figure 3.2

a) Mucocoele and involutional ectropion. Observe the bilateral lower lid fat protrusion, mid-face ptosis and eyelid laxity. There is a right lower lid medial ectropion and a right mucocoele. On the left there is early lower lid ectropion with punctal eversion and medialization. This patient had a sticky watery right eye and a watery left eye.

b) Paralytic ectropion with keratinization. Left chronic lower motor neurone facial palsy (normal corneal sensation). Lower lid hyperaemia and crusting secondary to exposure.

c) Involutional ectropion and lacrimal sac fistula. There is a right medial ectropion with a dry inferior punctum. There is also a fistula in the region of the lacrimal sac secondary to previous dacryocystitis.

d) Mechanical ectropion. Inflamed chalazion and lax eyelid syndrome causing right lateral ectropion in a man aged 44 years.

e) Tumour. Cicatricial medial ectropion from pericanalicular/medial lower lid basal cell carcinoma.

Face and periorbital examination

The lids and the lacrimal system should be addressed, as dual pathology may coexist (Figure 3.2).

TIP

Involutional ectropion and blocked nasolacrimal duct coexist in up to 10 per cent of elderly patients. Always syringe patients with lower lid ectropion.

Practice point: Epiphora and hypersecretion can coexist.

Medial canthal area assessment

Examine the medial canthal area. Feel for lumps and look for fistulas, inflammation and discharge. Locate the mass in relation to the medial canthal tendon. Be aware that not all masses in this area arise from the lacrimal sac (Figure 3.3).

TIP

Lacrimal sac swellings arise below the medial canthal tendon.

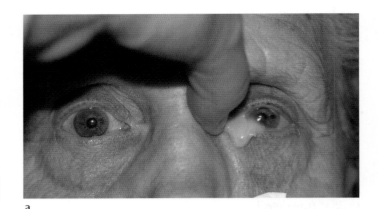

a

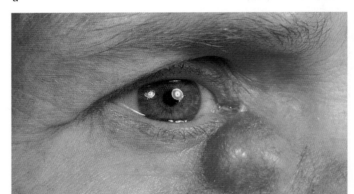

b

c

Figure 3.3

a) Mucocoele. Press over the lacrimal sac to see if there is an expressible mucocoele. Mucopurulent material can be expressed if the canaliculi and valve of Rosenmuller are healthy.
b) Chronic dacryocystitis with a large non-expressible mucocoele.
c) Blue coloured mass in the region of the lacrimal sac (below the medial canthal tendon). This patient had a *minimally* watering eye. This was a haemangioma extrinsic to the lacrimal sac.
d) Abscess arising from above the medial canthal tendon, unrelated to the lacrimal sac. The patient did *not* have a watering eye. She had an infected epidermoid cyst.

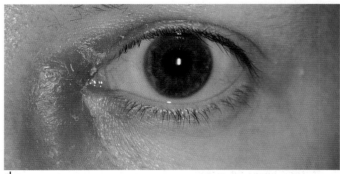

d

Anterior lamella shortening or vertical eyelid tightness

Examine the tightness of the anterior lamella (skin and muscle) to exclude causes of cicatricial ectropion. A short anterior lamella pulls the lid out and down. Check this by asking the patient to open the mouth widely and look up at the ceiling; if the anterior lamella is short, the ectropion will be exacerbated (Figure 3.4).

TIP

Look at the skin colour and texture – use the slit-lamp to look at fine detail.

Puncta and canaliculi

The puncta should face slightly towards the lacrimal lake. Confirm that all four puncta are present and open. Exclude stenosis and membranous occlusion. Examine the relative positions of the upper and lower puncta to each other and to the caruncle. Exclude conjunctivochalasis. Examine the caruncle.

Look for discharge from the puncta. If there is chronic red swelling medial to the puncta, exclude actinomycoses or fungal infection (Figure 3.5).

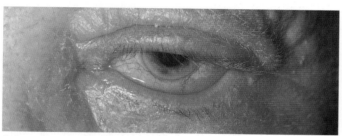

a

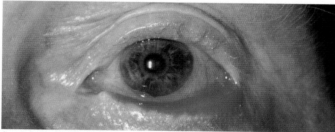

b

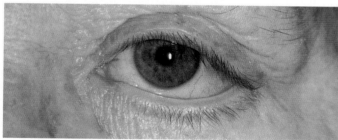

c

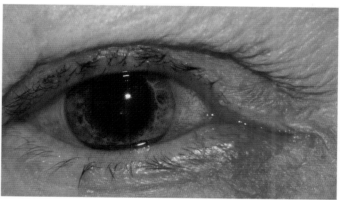

a

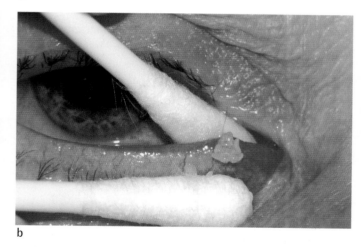

b

Figure 3.4

a) Allergy. Contact dermatitis from topical anti-glaucoma drops. Lid and cheek skin is red, dry, shiny and fissured. This is reversible by using preservative-free drops or substituting a trial of oral acetazoloamide.
b) Actinic skin changes cause predominantly lateral lower lid ectropion.
c) Lateral lower lid ectropion after lower lid blepharoplasty (skin and muscle excision) with uncorrected horizontal and lateral canthal laxity.

Figure 3.5

a) Chronic lower actinomycetes canaliculitis. A 'chalazion' type swelling is medial to the punctum. A true chalazion would be lateral.
b) Confirm canaliculitis by expressing yellow cheesy material from the canaliculus. This can be done simply by pressing on the swelling with a cotton bud or, if the material is not easily expressed, instilling topical anaesthesia and taking two cotton buds, one placed on each side of the canaliculus, to express the concretions or sulphur granules.

Diagrammatic record of periocular, eyelid and puncta assessment

Record the periorbital, eyelid and puncta findings diagrammatically (Figure 3.6). Superimpose lid malposition and any lumps over a simple line drawing of the lids, puncta and medial canthal tendon. Record the location of a mass in relation to the medial canthal tendon. Use reproducible symbols to represent the findings (Table 3.1).

R   L

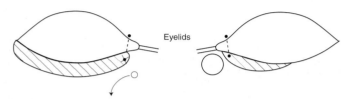

Eyelids

Figure 3.6

Diagrammatic record. Right complete lower lid ectropion with an occluded puncta and a fistula from the lacrimal sac. Left lower lid medial ectropion and a mucocoele. Published with permission from *Eye*.

Table 3.1 Examples of symbols used in diagrammatic record of periocular, eyelid and puncta assessment

Normal punctum	Small solid circle
Visible occluded punctum	Cross over small solid circle
No evidence of punctum	Cross over expected location
Stenosed punctum	Tiny dot surrounded by circle
Enlarged punctum (e.g. after three-snip)	Solid triangle
Medial displacement of punctum	Small arrow pointing medially
Fistula from sac	Small open circle with arrow

Assessment of involutional ectropion

Involutional ectropion can affect the entire lower lid, or exist only as mild punctal eversion seen on gentle lid closure. Involutional ectropion progresses from punctal eversion to involve the medial third, then the medial half of the lower eyelid. Eventually a total ectropion can develop (Figure 3.7).

The choice of surgery depends on:
1. The location and amount of ectropion
2. The medial canthal laxity (normal up to 2–3 mm)
3. The lateral canthal laxity (normal up to 2 mm)
4. The horizontal laxity (normal up to 6–8 mm); over 8 mm is lax.

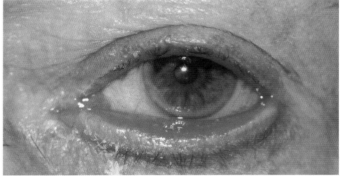

a

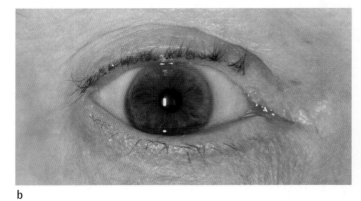

b

Figure 3.7

a) Complete ectropion. Lower lid tarsal eversion with secondary hyperaemia, keratinization and non-functioning 'dry' punctum.
b) Mild punctal eversion and medialization. The inferior punctum lies more medially than the upper. The normal inferior punctal resting position is just lateral to the upper punctum, next to the plica.

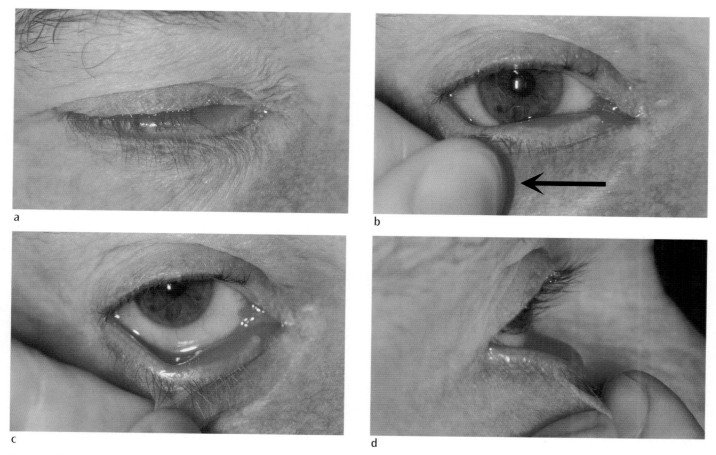

a

b

c

d

Figure 3.8

Same patient as Figure 3.7b.
a) Gentle eyelid closure reveals evident medial ectropion.
b) The lateral distraction test for medial canthal tendon laxity is assessed by pulling the lower lid laterally. The distance the lower punctum can be displaced along the horizontal line is recorded either in mm or graded (see Figure 3.11). Here the punctum cannot be pulled more than 1–2 mm laterally.
c) Pinch test for generalized horizontal laxity. Using the thumb and index finger, pull the lid firmly away from the globe and measure the distance between the lid and the eye.
d) Pinch test seen from the side. This lid has moderate laxity, approximately 10 mm.

These must be accurately assessed and recorded (Figures 3.8, 3.9).

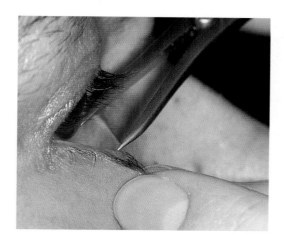

Figure 3.9

A calliper can be used to measure the distance from the posterior lid margin to the ocular surface accurately.

Horizontal laxity

The degree of horizontal eyelid laxity is estimated by the pinch test:

None	5 mm
Minimal	5–7 mm
Mild	8–9 mm
Moderate	10–12 mm
Severe	> 12 mm

The snap-back test is a dynamic test for lower lid tone. The lower lid is pulled down away from the globe then released. The speed with which the lid settles back against the globe is observed, as well as whether there is a short gap between the lid and globe once settled and before the first blink.

Medial canthal tendon laxity

The lower puncta should lie at the plica at rest and should remain there when the lid is pulled laterally (lateral distraction test). Up to 1–2 mm movement is normal in a young adult, and up to 3–4 mm in the elderly. If the punctum can be distracted beyond a line perpendicular to the medial limbus, the medial canthal tendon (MCT) is lax and stabilization, or other medial canthal surgery should be considered, when the lid is shortened horizontally. For examples, see Figure 3.10.

Medial canthal tendon laxity grading

This grading system is a simple way of recording MCT laxity. It is based on a visual scale in which the position of the punctum is recorded in relation to ocular surface landmarks, both at rest and with the lateral distraction test (Figure 3.11).

Steps:
1. Sit opposite the patient at a distance equivalent to arms' length and with eyes level.
2. Ask the patient to look at the bridge of your nose or glasses.
3. Ensure that you do not induce accommodative convergence by moving too close, and check that the patient doesn't have strabismus by doing a cover test.
4. Observe the resting position of the lower punctum

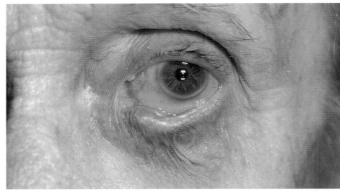

a

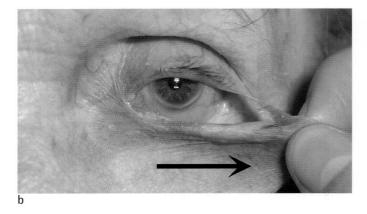

b

Figure 3.10

a)　Medial ectropion with punctal displacement both vertically and horizontally at rest. (Resting position +1).

b)　Lateral distraction test pulls the punctum beyond the mid-pupil (MCT laxity grade +6 to +7). Severe MCT laxity is present. This patient requires a large MCT stabilization or posterior fixation of the MCT at the same time as horizontal lid shortening.

Lateral distraction test

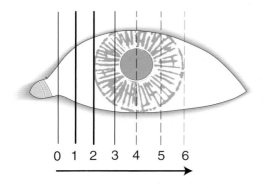

Figure 3.11

MCT laxity grading system.

in relation to the upper punctum, whether medial, in the same vertical line or lateral. The normal lower punctum resting position is situated at the lateral border of the plica, and this position is grade 0. Note that the plica extends laterally in its lower part.

5. Firmly pull the lower lid laterally (lateral distraction test) and observe the position along the horizontal axis that the punctum reaches. Record the finding in relation to the plica, medial limbus, pupillary line and lateral limbus.

Resting grade – lower punctal resting position:

−1	Punctal medialization
0	Normal
+1	Midway between the plica and medial limbus
+2	In line with the medial limbus
+3–+6	Beyond the medial limbus. These resting positions rarely occur

Grading MCT laxity – lateral distraction test:

0	No distraction at all
+1	Punctum reaches midpoint plica to medial limbus
+2	Punctum reaches medial limbus
+3	Punctum reaches midpoint medial limbus to pupil line
+4	Punctum reaches pupil line
+5	Punctum reaches midpoint pupil line to lateral limbus – rare
+6	Punctum reaches lateral limbus – extremely rare

Slit-lamp examination

Tear meniscus

Measure the vertical height of the tear meniscus prior to instillation of eyedrops. Record the finding diagrammatically and numerically.

The tear meniscus findings must be considered along with the other findings, such as dye retention test and syringing, and not alone.

TIP

When examining the tear meniscus, exclude blepharitis, dry eye and other external disease as a cause of hypersecretion and possible elevated tear meniscus.

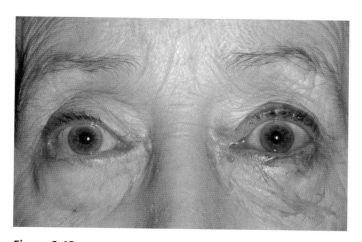

Figure 3.12

Fluorescein dye retention test. This patient had right dacryostenosis with mild functional epiphora and a left blocked nasolacrimal duct with marked epiphora. The FDRT confirms this asymmetry. At 3 minutes it is positive on the left and only just visible on the right.

Fluorescein dye tests

The fluorescein dye retention test (FDRT)

This is a semi-quantitative test of delayed or obstructed tear outflow, and is also called the fluorescein dye disappearance test (Figure 3.12). Instil one drop of fluorescein 2% into the unanaesthetized conjunctival sac. The amount of residual colour after 3 and 5 minutes in one or both eyes is noted and the intensity of residual dye graded. The test is positive if residual fluorescein is present. The dye normally drains down the system in this time. A strongly positive FDRT is found if obstruction is present. False negative findings may occur due to a large lacrimal sac or mucocoele, or a distal nasolacrimal duct block, where the dye can pool in the sac or duct.

FDRT findings: Grade using scale 0–4; 0 = no dye, 4 = all the dye.

Jones tests

For details of technique, see after syringing (Figure 3.16).

These are now rarely used, because the Jones I test has a high false negative rate, i.e. dye is not recovered when the system is in fact patent. They have been superseded by more accurate endoscopic versions, where fluorescein passing down the nasolacrimal duct into the nose is directly observed (see Figure 3.19).

The principles underlying the Jones I and II tests are, however, important, and should be understood. Jones tests are only performed to confirm and localize functional epiphora. They are not done if there is a complete obstruction on syringing.

Probing and irrigating the canaliculi and sac

Probing and irrigating (syringing) the proximal lacrimal drainage system is very informative. It can detect both the presence and site of partial or complete lacrimal outflow obstruction. It can reveal a small mucocoele by regurgitation of mucus. It must be done gently. If there is an obvious large mucocoele or dacryocystitis, only probe the canaliculi gently and do not irrigate, as inflating an inflamed lacrimal sac can be painful.

Care must be taken in the interpretation of soft and hard stops, as the hard stop (medial sac wall in lacrimal fossa) can feel softish. We therefore use the term 'bungie' feel for the soft stop of proximal common canalicular block and the term 'firm' stop for the medial sac wall and bone. The bungie feel can be accompanied by slight distortion of the medial canthal angle by the probe. A partial obstruction at the distal end of the common canaliculus can have a 'pop' feel as the cannula brushes past.

Irrigation is at a higher hydrostatic pressure than the normal tear outflow; therefore patients with functional epiphora from dacryostenosis may have apparently normal findings on irrigation, and lacrimal scintillography should be done. If this is not available, late erect dacryocystogram films help locate dacryostenosis.

Steps:
1. Make sure the patient is comfortable, with the head supported by a wall or head rest.
2. Dilate the lower punctum with a Nettleship dilator, first vertically and then horizontally, with the eyelid on stretch.
3. Very gently advance the cannula along the curve of the canaliculus, through the common canaliculus and into the lacrimal sac. Repeat via the upper punctum if the lower punctum is absent or there is canalicular obstruction (Figures 3.13, 3.14).

For upper punctum probing and irrigation, ask the patient to look down and laterally whilst stretching the canaliculus laterally and slightly everting the punctum with your finger. Topical anaesthesia is recommended, as syringing via the upper canaliculus is always more awkward.

If all the saline regurgitates from the same canaliculus, use the cannula to determine the canalicular patency. Measure the distance before the obstruction by placing the first finger and thumb on the probe close to the punctum, then withdrawing the probe and measuring the distance to its tip.

Compare the findings of intracanalicular and intrasac probing and irrigation to detect the presence of a partial distal common canalicular block (membranous) and dacryostenosis.

If the cannula cannot be advanced into the sac, observe carefully for any distortion of the medial canthal angle produced on attempted probing, consistent with proximal common canalicular block. This is the bungie feel or a soft stop.

TIP

Do not let the cannula kink the canaliculus and give a false impression of a block. Avoid this by keeping the eyelid on stretch and gently letting the cannula lead the hand rather than the hand pushing the cannula along the canaliculus.

TIP

Always stand on the side that is being probed and irrigated.

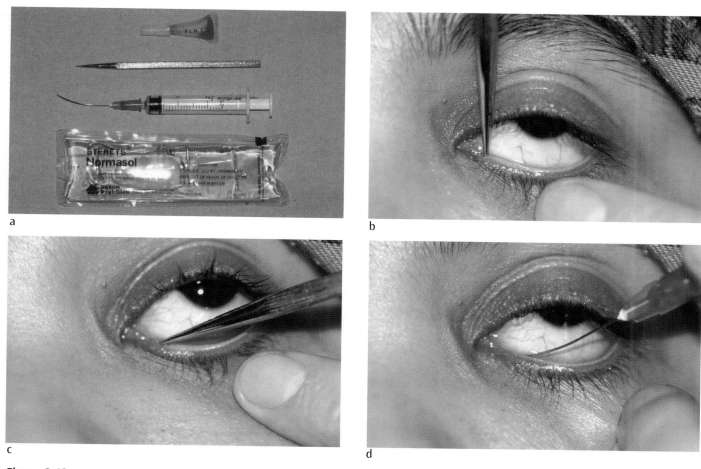

Figure 3.13

a)　Syringing equipment:
　　(i)　Fluorescein
　　(ii)　Nettleship dilator
　　(iii)　2 ml syringe with 26 g disposable lacrimal cannula (slightly curved)
　　(iv)　Normal saline.
b)　Ask the patient to look upwards – topical anaesthesia is not mandatory if the eye is not touched. Pull the lower lid down and laterally to straighten the lower canaliculus and evert the punctum away from the ocular surface. Hold the lid in this position throughout. Dilate the punctum and vertical part of the canaliculus (ampulla) with the Nettleship dilator.
c)　Once in the ampulla, change direction of the Nettleship by 90° to enter and dilate the proximal horizontal part of the canaliculus.
d)　Gentle irrigation.

Recording the findings on syringing

The findings are recorded on a skeleton line drawing showing the canaliculi, common canaliculus, lacrimal sac and nasolacrimal duct. An arrow over the lower canaliculus indicates that probing and irrigation were via the lower canaliculus. Similarly, an arrow over the upper canaliculus indicates that it was via that canaliculus. An arrow at the lower end of the nasolacrimal duct indicates that saline drained freely into the patient's throat.

TIP

Develop a mental image of the findings from probing and syringing, and record this on an outline of the canaliculi, sac and nasolacrimal duct.

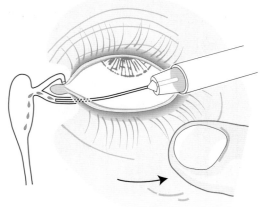

a

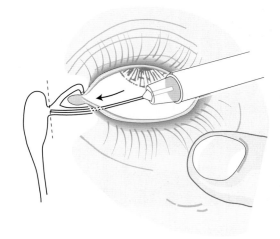

b

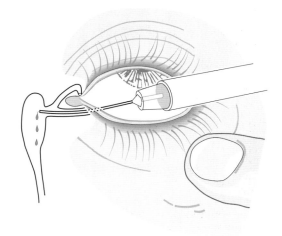

c

Figure 3.14

a)　Gently insert the lacrimal cannula, first vertically then horizontally with the curve of the cannula as shown. Advance slowly into the mid-canaliculus and irrigate approximately 0.5 ml. Observe whether there is any regurgitation via the same canaliculus, the upper punctum or both, and whether the patient swallows/detects fluid in the throat. This is the *intra-canalicular irrigation*.

b)　Advance the cannula extremely gently. Feel for any slight give ('pop') between the common canaliculus and sac indicative of a partial (membranous) block or valve effect (valve of Rosenmuller).

c)　Gently advance to the medial wall of the sac (firm feel, sometimes tender) then withdraw back into the sac by 1–2 mm and irrigate 0.25–0.5 ml. This is *intra-sac irrigation*. Observe again whether there is any regurgitation or free flow to the throat.

Regurgitation via one or both canaliculi is shown by a reversed arrow. If this was only slight and some saline reached the nose, the arrow can be broken, indicating functional nasolacrimal duct stenosis. Complete nasolacrimal duct block is indicated by a large cross and 'nil' written at the lower end of the duct.

A complete common canalicular block is shown by a solid vertical line, and a partial (membranous) block by a broken vertical line.

Individual canalicular findings, including the length of patent canaliculus, are recorded. If the canaliculus cannot be probed, it is written as a dotted 'unknown' line (Figure 3.15).

TIP

If you find a common canalicular block, there may be a normal sac and nasolacrimal duct beyond which cannot be assessed or commented upon.

The Jones tests – technique and interpretation

The Jones tests are dye tests for functional epiphora where it is known from syringing that the lacrimal drainage system is patent (Figure 3.16). They are used in conjunction with the FDRT, probing and irrigation, and can help differentiate hypersecretion and epiphora.

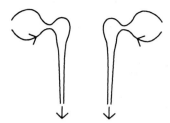

Bilateral normal syringing and sac
probing via lower canaliculus

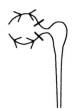

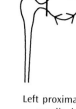

Right upper and lower
distal canalicular block

Left proximal common
canalicular block

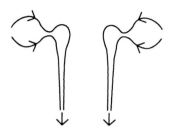

Bilateral normal syringing and sac probing
via both upper and lower canaliculus

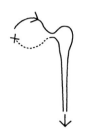

Right lower punctum
absent

3 mm

3 mm

Nil

Left upper and lower
proximal canalicular block

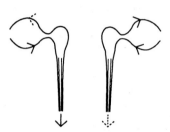

Functional epiphora from nasolacrimal
duct stenosis. Left more marked than right

Mucous
+

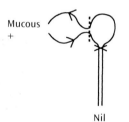

Nil   Nil

Right expressible
mucocoele

Left non-expressible
mucocoele

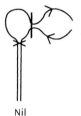

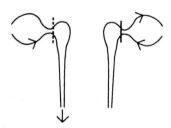

Right **partial** and left **complete** distal
common canalicular block

2 mm

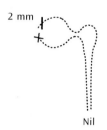

Nil

Right complete upper
canalicular proximal block,
and occluded lower punctum

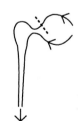

Left upper canalicular
partial distal block

Figure 3.15

Diagrams of findings on
syringing.

TIP

*The Jones tests are of no value if you know the lacrimal
system is blocked to syringing. You should irrigate the
system first.*

Steps for Jones I test

1. Patient is seated, with the eyes not anaesthetized to
    allow normal blinking.
2. Decongest/anaesthetize the nasal mucosa.

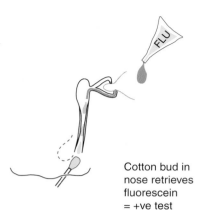

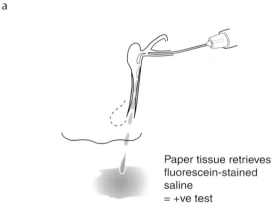

Cotton bud in
nose retrieves
fluorescein
= +ve test

a

Paper tissue retrieves
fluorescein-stained
saline
= +ve test

b

Figure 3.16

a) Diagram showing positive Jones I test.
b) Diagram showing positive Jones II test.

3. Instil guttae fluorescein 2% into the conjunctival
    sac.
4. Place a cotton bud/tip in the nose below the inferior
    turbinate (IT) as far as the nasolacrimal duct
    opening (1 cm behind the anterior end of the IT).
5. The test is positive if dye is found on the cotton
    bud.

A positive Jones I test (dye recovered from nose)
indicates nasolacrimal drainage and is of little value,
since you already know if there is anatomical patency
from syringing. The epiphora could be from
hypersecretion or a functional epiphora.

If the Jones I test is negative (no dye is recovered from
the nose) an obstruction of the nasolacrimal system may
be present and a Jones II test is recommended.

The Jones I test has an unacceptably high false negative
rate (22 per cent), as the dye transit times are influenced
by patient position, blink rate, gravity, fluorescein
volume, nasal floor and IT anatomy.

Modifications of the Jones I test

1. *Oropharynx dye appearance test.* This is useful for
    infants, where syringing requires sedation or general
    anaesthesia. Instil guttae fluorescein 2% into the
    conjunctival sac and use a blue light to look at the
    oropharynx for fluorescein, at intervals, for up to 30
    minutes. Only one side should be tested at a time for
    accurate localization.
2. *Taste saccharin test.* Instil 0.4 ml of 2% saccharin
    drops into the conjunctival sac. The average time
    from instillation to taste is 31/2 minutes, with 90 per
    cent of patients tasting by 15 minutes. It is best to
    do one side at a time.
3. *Endonasal dye tests.* These are increasingly replacing
    the Jones I test.

Steps for the Jones II test

1. Wash out any residual fluorescein from the
    conjunctival sac with guttae saline.
2. Instil topical anaesthesia.
3. Patient is seated with head tilted forwards.
4. Do a transcanalicular irrigation with saline. Ask the
    patient to blow or spit the fluid onto a paper tissue –
    look to see if residual fluorescein from the original
    Jones I test is present (a positive result).
5. A positive test suggests the dye reached the lacrimal
    sac but, in the presence of a narrowed nasolacrimal
    duct, required the syringing pressure to force it
    down.

A positive Jones II confirms anatomical patency with a
high-pressure wash-out of fluorescein. There is
physiological or anatomical partial block below the sac,
and surgery is indicated, depending on the patient's
symptoms.

If both the Jones I and Jones II tests are negative, high
grade functional stenosis is present and surgery is
indicated.

If clear fluid is irrigated in the Jones II test (negative finding), this indicates that fluorescein did not get into the lacrimal sac with the Jones I test. There may be eyelid malposition, lacrimal pump failure (paralytic), or punctal or canalicular stenosis.

TIP

Only proceed to the Jones II test if the Jones I test is negative – i.e. suggests delayed outflow.

Practice point: Only do the Jones tests if you are sure you understand their principles and interpretation. Consider doing an endoscopic dye test, magnified and directly viewed.

The information obtained from the Jones I and II tests can be obtained from careful periocular and eyelid examination, the FDRT, gentle probing and irrigation, endonasal dye tests and nuclear lacrimal scintillography.

Part B: Nasal examination

Principles of nasal endoscopy

Rigid nasal endoscopy is used in lacrimal disease for diagnosis, treatment, and video recording of findings.

Diagnosis

An endonasal examination is performed to exclude anatomical variations and pathology that contribute to lacrimal system obstruction or may interfere with surgery.

Approximately 85 per cent of patients with acquired nasolacrimal duct obstruction have radiological (computer tomography) evidence of sinus disease or rhinological abnormality such as septal deviation, compared to just over 60 per cent of control subjects. Many of these findings can be detected by endoscopy.

Equipment

1. *Nasal speculum and headlight.* This provides a poor view of the region in the nose adjacent to the lacrimal sac and duct.
2. *Rigid nasal endoscope with light source.*

The rigid endoscope was developed by Professor H. H. Hopkins in the mid-1970s, and is a popular tool in medicine. It is a small-diameter rod and lens system that provides a wide viewing angle with a bright image.

Advances in rigid endoscopy have arisen as a result of improved techniques in minimally invasive functional endoscopic sinus surgery (FESS). FESS was a technique initially developed by Professor Messerklinger in Austria in the 1980s for the diagnosis and management of patients with paranasal sinus disease.

A 4 mm or 2.7 mm diameter, 0° viewing angle rigid Hopkins endoscope attached to a fibre optic or hand-held light source provides a clearly illuminated and magnified view (up to 16×) of the nasal space, useful both for endonasal lacrimal surgery and for office nasal examination. The 4 mm version is the more robust endoscope, although the 2.7 mm has the advantage that it can be used routinely for adult nasal evaluation without nasal decongestion, and kept for endonasal monitoring of paediatric syringe and probing.

Other viewing angles available include the 30°, 45° and 70° endoscopes, which enable the surgeon to look sideways. The 30° and 45° endoscopes are suitable for endonasal lacrimal surgery, whilst the 70º version is more useful for sinus surgery where, for instance, the surgeon wants to look into the maxillary sinus. There is a reduction in illumination with decreasing endoscope diameter and length and with increasing viewing angle (Figure 3.17).

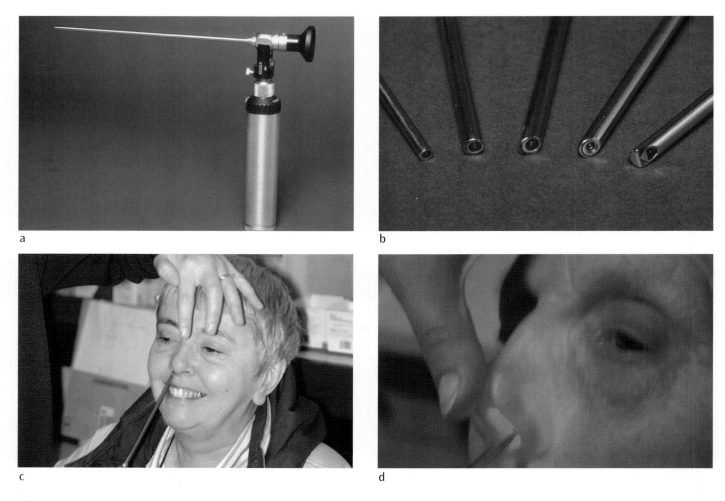

Figure 3.17

a) 4 mm 0° rigid Hopkins endoscope on an otoscope handle.
b) Different endoscopes. Left to right: 2.7 mm 0°, 4 mm 0°, 4 mm 30°, 4 mm 45°, 4 mm 70°.
c) Outpatient nasal endoscopy showing comfortable patient.
d) Examiner's thumb on tip of patient's nose and endoscope directed towards the lacrimal sac region.

Remote viewing with a video camera attachment is only required for teaching, research and for a permanent record. Direct viewing provides better acuity.

Nasal preparation for endoscopy

The nasal mucosa should be vasoconstricted for easy access and a clear view. The inferior turbinate, in particular, contains submucous erectile venous sinusoids, which swell and compromise the view unless it is decongested.

Decongestants:
1. Guttae phenylephrine 2.5 or 10% (applied on cotton buds placed in the nasal space). NB: Avoid use of 10% in patients with hypertension and in the elderly.
2. Guttae oxymetazoline or zylomatazoline 0.05% or 0.1% is used for hypertensive patients (also applied on cotton buds).
3. Cophenylcaine Forte nasal spray (also contains topical anaesthesia, lignocaine). This is the best option but will also reach the pharynx and numb it; therefore the patient should be told to avoid hot drinks for 1 hour afterwards.

If cotton buds soaked with vasoconstrictor are used, they are directed up towards the middle turbinate and left in the nose for 3 minutes. The fluid does not reach the pharynx and numb it.

Nasal endoscopy technique

Nasal preparation is as above.

Patient preparation

The patient is seated, as still and relaxed as possible, breathing gently through the mouth and avoiding neck hyperextension. The examiner can stand if remote viewing is used, or sit for direct viewing.

Explain to the patient that the endoscope is a thin torch with which to look inside the nose, and that it will not hurt.

Examining the nasal space

Coat the endoscope tip with anti-fog solution. Ultrastop® or Fred®. A Steret® is equally effective. The endoscope tip can be dipped in warm (not hot) water if the room temperature is cool.

Right-handed examiner. Lightly evert the tip of the patient's nose with the left thumb and balance the rest of the hand on the patient's forehead for stabilization. Enter the nasal vestibule, avoiding the vascular plexus of Kisselbach inferior medially, which can bleed if touched by the endoscope. Keep the axis of the endoscope parallel to the septum and inspect the anterior nasal space.

The tip of the nose no longer needs to be held everted. Advance into the nasal cavity in a systematic way. There are three steps to examining areas of interest without taking the endoscope out:

1. Inspect the floor and inferior meatus, inferior turbinate and lower septum
2. Direct the endoscope above the inferior turbinate to examine the lacrimal ridge (maxillary line), the anterior part of the middle turbinate and the middle meatus

3. Direct the endoscope up to the neck of the middle turbinate and medial to the middle turbinate.

Try to avoid making the patient sneeze. Do not direct the endoscope too high and anterior towards the 'sneeze' spot in the nasal roof.

Normal nasal anatomy

Straight septum and normal turbinates (Figure 3.18).

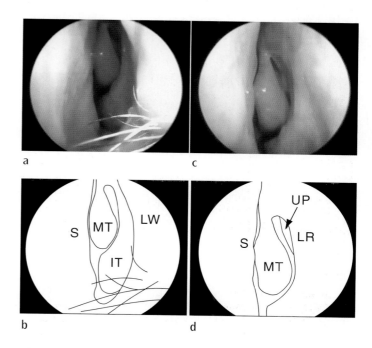

Figure 3.18

a) Endoscopic view of left anterior nasal space from the vestibule. The septum (on left) is straight. The inferior turbinate is seen on the right, inferiorly, and the anterior aspect of the middle turbinate superiorly.
b) Key diagram for (a); S = septum, MT = middle turbinate, LW = lateral wall, IT = inferior turbinate.
c) The endoscope has been advanced above the inferior turbinate to examine the lacrimal ridge and view the middle turbinate. The uncinate process is just visible in the middle meatus, lateral to the middle turbinate. The middle turbinate looks normal, although it may be partially pneumatized. Note its lateral concavity and the wide middle meatus.
d) Key diagram for (c); S = septum, MT = middle turbinate, UP = uncinate process, LR = lacrimal ridge.

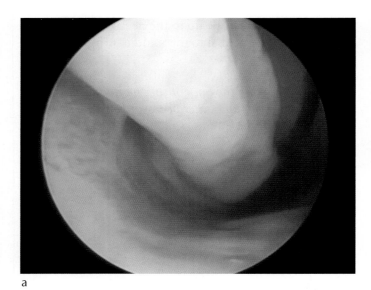

a

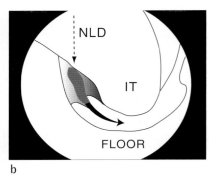

b

Figure 3.19

a) Right inferior meatus with fluorescein clearly visible.
b) Key diagram; NLD = nasolacrimal duct, IT = inferior turbinate.

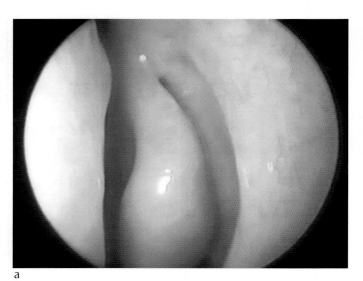

a

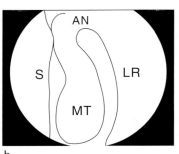

b

Figure 3.20

a) Left paradoxical middle turbinate. The lateral mucosal surface is in close contact with the mucosa of the lateral nasal wall. The middle meatus is narrow. An agger nasi (pneumatized anterior ethmoid cell) forming a bulge anterior to the insertion of the middle turbinate on the lateral nasal wall is present. This would be encountered at DCR surgery because it lies between the lacrimal sac and the nose.
b) Key diagram for (a);
    S = septum,
    AN = agger nasi,
    MT = middle turbinate,
    LR = lacrimal ridge.
c) Right large concha bullosa. This middle turbinate is entirely pneumatized. The medial and lateral mucosal surfaces of the turbinate are touching the septal and lateral wall mucosa.
d) Key diagram for (c);
    LR = lacrimal ridge,
    MT = middle turbinate,
    S = septum.

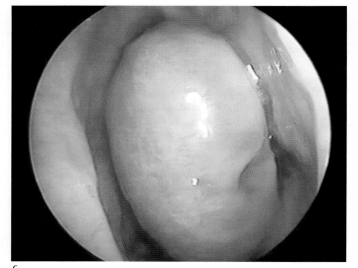

c

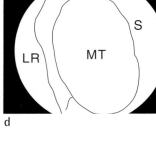

d

Endoscopic Jones I test

The standard Jones test has been described. For the endoscopic test, instead of using a cotton bud, an endoscope is used to view the floor and inferior meatus. Look for fluorescein emerging from the opening of the nasolacrimal duct in the inferior meatus. The fluorescein drains down the remaining distance of the lateral nasal wall, then posteriorly along the floor. The use of a blue cobalt light has been described as an aid in detecting fluorescein, but is not usually necessary in order to visualize it. A study has shown that the endoscopic Jones I test is six times more sensitive than the conventional Jones I test in detecting fluorescein in the nose (Figure 3.19).

Middle turbinate variations

The normal middle turbinate curves away from the lateral nasal wall – it has a straight to slightly concave lateral contour when viewed by anterior nasal endoscopy.

Anatomical variations may initially confuse the inexperienced endoscopist and therefore need to be recognized (Figure 3.20).

> **Common middle turbinate variations:**
> * Paradoxical
> * Elongated
> * Anterior extending
> * Concha bullosa (pneumatized).

> **Rarer middle turbinate variations:**
> * Bifid
> * Duplicated
> * Lateralized (atrophic and collapsed laterally).

When the lateral surface of the middle turbinate is close to or in direct contact with the lateral nasal wall, there is an increased risk of adhesion (synaechiae) after lacrimal surgery. Synaechiae between the middle turbinate and lateral nasal wall can occlude the dacryocystorhinostomy ostium to cause surgical failure.

If the middle turbinate is large and extended anteriorly, it can interfere with correct Jones tube placement. It is sometimes necessary to correct the abnormality by a partial turbinectomy. This should not be done routinely!

Septal deviation

The septum ideally lies in the middle of the nasal cavity, dividing it into two sides. Most patients have a degree of nasal septal deviation where the septum lies to one side of the midline in part or all of its course, making the nasal space relatively narrow on one side. Mild asymmetry does not affect breathing, although a severely deviated septum can do so. Septal deviation is usually congenital; a history should be taken alluding to any possible traumatic cause.

> **A narrowed nasal space makes the following more difficult:**
> * Nasal examination
> * Endonasal surgery, including placement of Jones bypass tubes
> * Retrieval of silicone dacryocystorhinostomy tubes.

With increased vasoconstriction and practice, these difficulties diminish. Traumatic or severe septal deviation may require a submucosal resection (SMR) prior to endonasal lacrimal surgery. A narrowed nasal space should be identified before surgery and a decision made as to whether an SMR is necessary, particularly if a Jones bypass tube is planned, as its aftercare requires easy endonasal access (Figure 3.21).

Uncinate process variations

The uncinate process can extend anteriorly or medially and be visible in the middle meatus. It may also touch the middle turbinate (Figure 3.22).

TIP

During endonasal dacryocystorhinostomy, thin uncinate bone can be encountered lying medial to the lacrimal bone when the lacrimal fossa is opened.

> **Uncinate process variations:**
> * Medially bent
> * Anteriorly rotated
> * Enlarged
> * Combination of above.

Practice point: Expect surprises when you look in the nose!

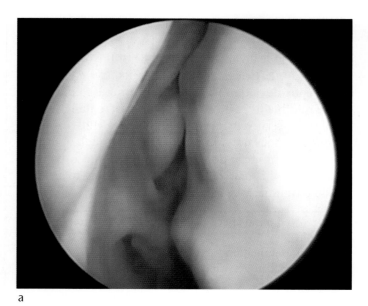

a

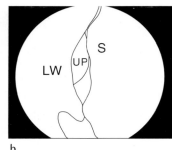

b

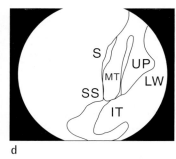

d

c

Figure 3.21

Nasal asymmetry.
a) Right narrowed nasal space with septal deviation. The swelling just posterior to the lacrimal ridge could be the middle turbinate or a medially bent uncinate process. It is necessary to advance the endoscope to elaborate the anatomy.
b) Key diagram for (a); LW = lateral wall, UP = uncinate process, S = septum.
c) Left wide nasal space (same patient) with nasal septal spur. A medially bent uncinate process is visible lateral to the middle meatus.
d) Key diagram for (c); SS = septal spur, MT = middle turbinate, IT = inferior turbinate, UP = uncinate process, LR = lacrimal ridge.

Nasal pathology

Symptoms of nasal disease can be mild, including nasal obstruction or discharge, or even non-existent. Exclude obvious nasal pathology, including evidence of previous nasal surgery. Computer tomography may be required in addition to rigid nasal endoscopy (Figures 3.23–3.29).

Nasal pathology:
1. Rhinosinusitis
    ● Allergic
    ● Infective
    ● Non-allergic/non-infective
    ● Polyps
2. Granulomatous disease
    ● Wegener's granulomatosis
    ● Sarcoidosis
    ● Tuberculosis

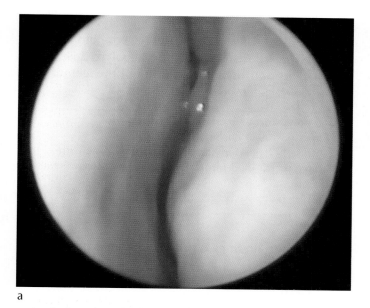

a

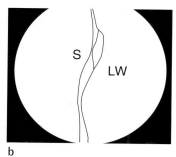

b

c

d

Figure 3.22

a) Left nasal space examination. Entry – narrowed space. A 'middle turbinate' is visible in the distance.

b) Key diagram for (a); S = septum, LW = lateral wall.

c) Further advancing to the neck of the middle turbinate, the lateral wall structures are now clearly visible. The inferior turbinate is out of view and the uncinate process is bent or rotated medially.

d) Key diagram for (c); S = septum, MT = middle turbinate, UP = uncinate process, LR = lacrimal ridge.

3. Benign paranasal tumour
    - Osteoma
    - Inverted papilloma (behaves aggressively)
4. Malignant paranasal tumour
    - Squamous cell carcinoma
    - Adenocarcinoma
    - Lymphoma
    - Secondary

5. Lacrimal sac tumour extending into nasal space (uncommon compared to paranasal tumours)
6. Previous lateral rhinotomy or FESS surgery.

Practice point: If nasal pathology is found, seek the advice of an otolaryngologist who specializes in rhinology.

Examine the mucosal appearance to exclude rhinitis; in addition to infection (acute viral rhinitis and chronic bacterial rhinitis) there are several other causes:

Appearance of mucosa	Type of rhinitis
Pale grey/bluish, boggy	Allergic
Red and oedematous	Inflammation
Dry and crusty	Atrophic
Swollen red with pale ischaemic damage	Medicamentosa
Engorged inferior turbinate, lots of clear watery rhinorrhoea	Vasomotor
Yellow, dry patches of exudate	Chronic bacterial
Red with stringy scant mucus	Acute viral

obstruction. These include loss of smell and a watery nose. Extensive polyps can expand the ethmoid sinuses to cause hypertelorism. Antrochoanal polyps arise from the maxillary antrum and appear out of the natural ostium on the lateral nasal wall.

> **Nasal polyps occur in several diseases:**
> * Small polyps in chronic rhinosinusitis
> * Diffuse polyposis in sinobranchial syndrome with acetylsalicylic acid intolerance and hyperactive airways disease
> * Diffuse polyposis associated with cystic fibrosis.

Nasal polyps are soft, pedunculated, vascular growths seen hanging down between the middle turbinate and the lateral nasal wall. They can range from solitary, multiple or diffuse, and are either an asymptomatic finding on nasal endoscopy or cause symptoms of nasal

Recording the findings on nasal examination

Record the endoscopy findings on a skeleton diagram showing the key features on the lateral nasal wall and the septum.

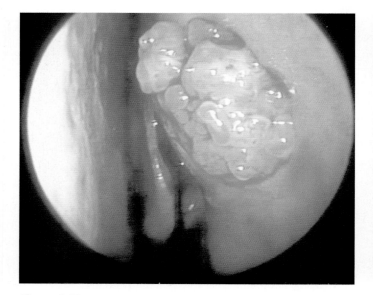

Figure 3.23

Lacrimal sac tumour (carcinoma) occluding the healed dacryocystorhinostomy ostium.

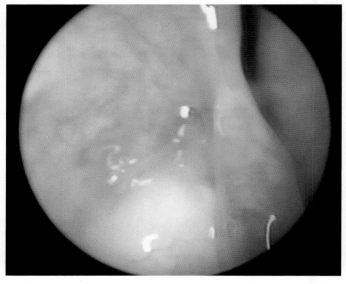

Figure 3.24

Right polyp hanging down between middle turbinate and lateral wall.

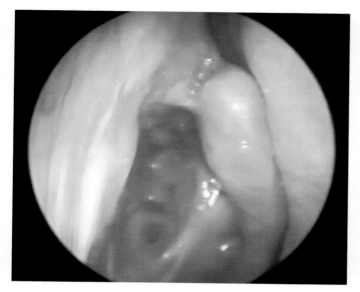

Figure 3.25

Right post-operative appearance after lateral rhinotomy for maxillary tumour. The nasolacrimal duct was excised with the tumour. The middle turbinate is recognizable, but reduced surgically.

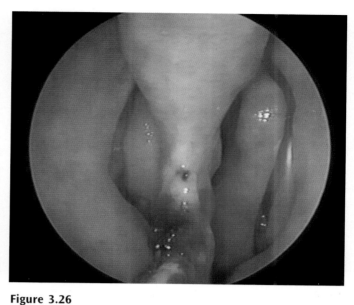

Figure 3.26

Bilateral view of idiopathic septal hole with normal lateral nasal wall structures. There is crusting secondary to dryness from abnormal air currents. The light seen on the right lateral nasal wall is a light pipe in the lower part of the lacrimal sac, prior to endonasal lacrimal surgery.

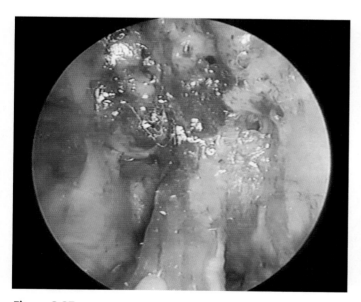

Figure 3.27

Wegener's granulomatosis. Bilateral extensive septal destruction. The mucosa is crusting and angry looking. There are no identifiable landmarks apart from the right and left lateral nasal walls.

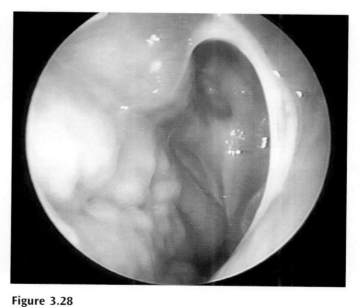

Figure 3.28

Sarcoidosis. Left middle/posterior nasal space showing destruction of normal architecture, pale lumpy submucosal cobblestones, inflammation and chronic rhinosinusitis.

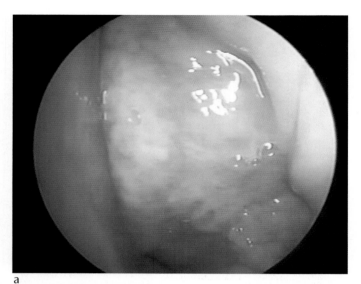

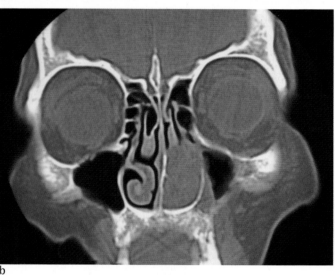

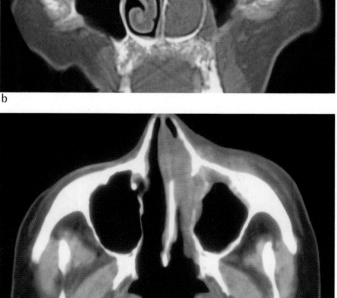

Figure 3.29

a) Tumour blocking left nasal space. This patient presented with a 6-month history of epiphora and more recent nasal obstruction. An incisional biopsy confirmed a malignant high grade B cell lymphoma.

b), c) Computer tomography coronal (b) and axial (c) views demonstrating the tumour within the left nasal space and nasolacrimal duct, and extending into the maxilla.

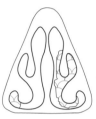

R   L

Normal nasal anatomy

Bilateral nasal polyps (L > R)

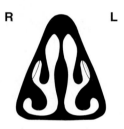

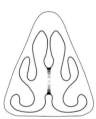

Left narrow nasal space with deviated septum and concha bullosa of middle turbinate

Hole in septum

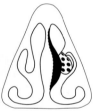

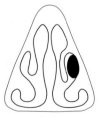

Left prominent (rotated) uncinate process and elongated middle turbinate

Previous left lateral rhinotomy – maxillectomy

Figure 3.30

The findings of endoscopic nasal examination are recorded diagrammatically on a skeleton line drawing showing the nasal space with septum and lateral wall structures. These are examples of pre-operative nose findings.

Part C: Radiology

Radiological examinations include:

1. Dacryocystography (DCG)
2. Nuclear lacrimal scintigraphy/radionuclide dacryocystography/nuclear lacrimal scan
3. Computer tomography (CT)
4. Magnetic resonance imaging (MRI) – rarely required.

Ancillary radiological investigations help confirm the site of stenosis or obstruction, confirm functional tear drainage delay, and demonstrate paranasal pathology. Tests are complementary, and more than one test may be necessary.

It is desirable to have either a dacrycystogram or lacrimal scintigraphy prior to dacryocystorhinostomy. DCG is indicated if there is a proven block on syringing, whilst scintigraphy is useful in assessing the site of delayed transit (functional epiphora) when syringing is patent. Both tests can be done, as they provide complementary information when planning surgery. CT scanning is only recommended in some patients where tumour, trauma or sinus disease is suspected.

TIP

If there is an obvious clinical diagnosis of regurgitating mucocoele, a DCG is not necessary. If there is obvious clinical acute dacryocystitis, a DCG is best avoided as it would be very painful for the patient.

Dacryocystography

This is injection of radio-opaque fluid into either the lower or the upper canaliculus and taking magnified images.

DCG enables an accurate assessment of the anatomy of the canaliculi, sac and nasolacrimal duct. It is good for determining the site of stenosis or obstruction, and is particularly useful in distinguishing between post-sac and pre-sac stenosis. It outlines diverticulae and fistulae, and shows intra-sac pathology (dacryoliths or tumour) and sac size. It also helps define the cause of failed lacrimal surgery.

Although semi-functional information may be obtained by late erect views (> 10 minutes after intra-canalicular injection), nuclear lacrimal scanning (scintigraphy) is better for function.

> **Intubation dacryocystography: procedure**
> - Patient is supine
> - Use topical anaesthesia
> - Dilate punctum (lower is fine)
> - Insert a fine cannula with attached 2 ml syringe containing contrast medium
> - Inject intra-canalicularly under pressure
> - Take films at approximately 30 s, 2 min, 5 min, and later erect films (at 12–15 min).

It is best to do bilateral simultaneous DCGs, as this gives relative functional information. Digital subtraction DCG provides a high quality image (Figure 3.31).

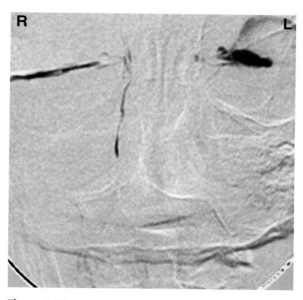

Figure 3.31

Bilateral digital subtraction DCG in a patient with left epiphora, 14 minutes after injection. Left complete block at the sac/duct junction, very small sac, and reflux into the conjunctival sac. Right bony spur at upper end of nasolacrimal duct; otherwise anatomically within normal limits. Lacrimal scintigraphy would provide little additional information. This patient needs a left dacryocystorhinostomy.

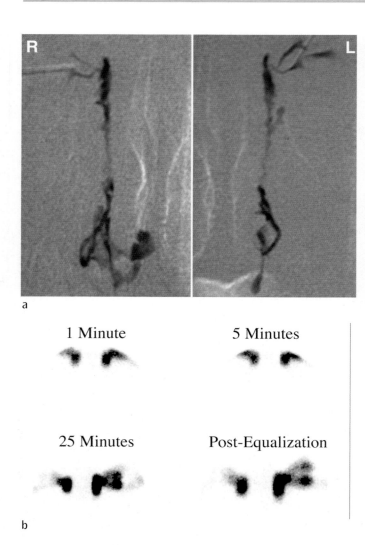

a

1 Minute   5 Minutes

25 Minutes   Post-Equalization

b

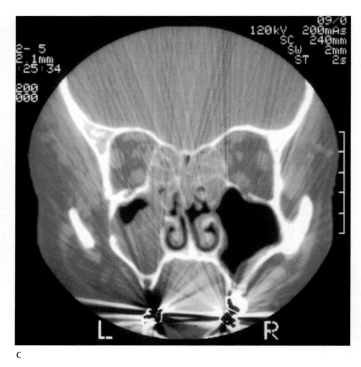

c

Figure 3.32

Comparative findings from a) digital subtraction DCG, b) nuclear lacrimal scintigraphy and c) coronal CT scan. This patient has bilateral functional epiphora. Syringing is patent with some regurgitation, there is no ocular surface disease, and no lid margin malposition or abnormal puncta. The tear menisci are elevated and FDRT moderately positive.

a)   The DCG shows patent but narrowed ragged mid-nasolacrimal ducts. On the left there is a diverticulum from the upper part of the nasolacrimal duct, below which the duct is irregular and narrowed.

b)   Lacrimal scintigraphy shows bilateral functional obstruction with no tracer detected in the nose on either side.

c)   Coronal CT scan of orbits and sinuses showing bilateral ethmoid and right maxillary sinus polyposis. The functional nasolacrimal duct obstruction is post-sac, in the mid- to upper part of the duct. This patient needs bilateral dacryocystorhinostomy.

TIP

Always look at the DCG yourself. You may spot something subtle that the radiologist has not noticed.

CT-DCG has been advocated by some surgeons, but is not used much. Separate CT and DCG are more informative.

Nuclear lacrimal scintigraphy

This uses a radiotracer (technitium 99m pertechnetate), which is very easily detectable and therefore only minute doses are required. One-sixtieth the dose of that used in a bone scan is required (approximately 5–10 mega

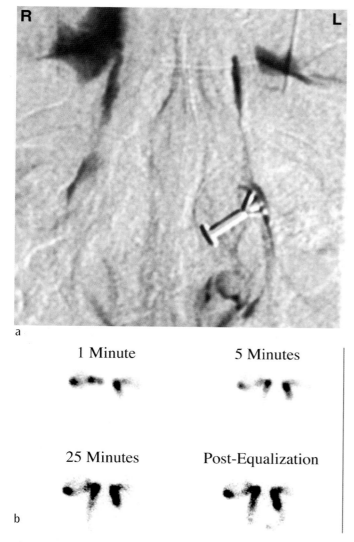

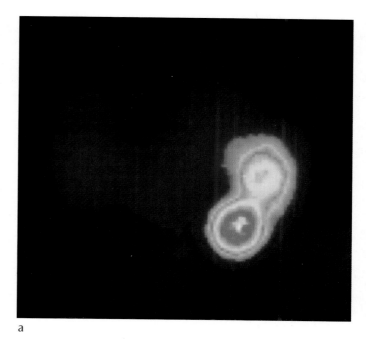

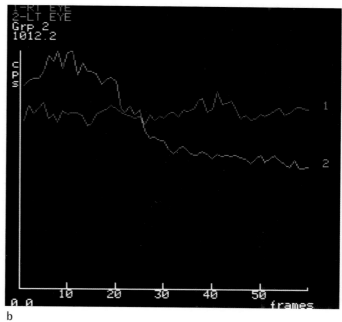

Figure 3.33

Comparative findings: a) digital subtraction DCG; b) lacrimal scintigraphy. This patient has epiphora right > left. Periorbital, lid and ocular surface findings are normal. The right tear meniscus is elevated and the fluorescein dye retention test (FDRT) strongly positive.

a) Bilateral digital subtraction DCG view 18 minutes after injection shows regurgitation of contrast media onto the conjunctival sac, mainly on the right, with a narrowed mid-nasolacrimal duct. The left clearly shows the sac, and the nasolacrimal duct is narrowed. Both sides show anatomical patency.

b) Lacrimal scintigraphy shows on the right side delayed appearance of tracer activity at the sac/duct junction, with retention of tracer activity in the conjunctival sac (pseudo-canalicular appearance). The left side shows only slightly abnormal tracer activity at mid- to lower duct. There is a nose ring.

The complementary findings confirm right significant functional epiphora needing dacryocystorhinostomy.

Figure 3.34

Nuclear lacrimal scintigraphy. a) Colour acquisition studies with b) region of interest analysis. This patient with functional epiphora has effectively no clearance from the right lacrimal system. The colour image from the right side at 30 minutes shows considerable residual retention of activity. The activity curves show reasonable drainage from the left side, but virtually none from the right side (semi-quantitative data). This patient needs a right dacryocystorhinostomy.

becquerels (MBq)/eye), instilled into the conjunctival sac as a drop, with the patient sitting next to the scintillation (gamma) camera. Tracer activity within the lacrimal system is recorded at intervals through the pinhole collimeter. Images are taken immediately, then at 5, 10, 15, 20 and 25 minutes for qualitative analysis. Quantitative, region-of-interest analysis is available, which will give percentage drainage with time. It is a safe physiological method for evaluating lacrimal drainage. No topical anaesthesia is required, and normal blinking is allowed.

It is only useful in those patients whose lacrimal system is patent to syringing. DCG is preferred if there is a complete obstruction.

The areas of interest on lacrimal scintigraphy are:
- Pre-sac
- Sac/nasolacrimal duct junction
- Mid-duct
- (Infra-duct).

Delay may occur at any of these sites. If there is pre-sac delay, suspect lid *or* canalicular disease. Note that the canaliculi are not seen with scintigraphy; instead the tracer is detected between the upper and lower lids. This can initially be mistaken for the outline of the upper and lower canaliculi – 'pseudocanaliculi'.

Correlation of the anatomical study (DCG) and functional study (lacrimal scintigraphy) may be necessary in planning surgery. A CT scan is also informative in certain cases.

Otolaryngologists evaluate their patients using coronal and axial CT with bone windows before functional endoscopic sinus surgery. Lacrimal surgeons are increasingly realizing the value of CT scanning in the evaluation of their patients, since it can show rhinosinus pathology and clearly demonstrate bony anatomy, particularly after trauma.

Functional epiphora

Some patients have nasolacrimal duct narrowing without complete obstruction, causing epiphora. DCG and lacrimal scintigraphy are complementary in their assessment (Figures 3.32, 3.33).

Lacrimal scintigraphy quantitative studies are helpful in functional epiphora, but not in general use (Figure 3.34).

Practice point: The coexistence of sinus disease and epiphora is higher than expected by chance, suggesting that the nasolacrimal duct and rhinosinus mucosas share a common inflammatory process.

Bibliography

Periorbital, lid and lacrimal system assessment:

Conway, S. T. (1994). Evaluation and management of 'functional' nasolacrimal blockage: results of a survey of the American Society of Ophthalmic Plastic and Reconstructive Surgery. *Ophth. Plastic Reconstr. Surg.*, 10, 185–7.

Flack, A. (1979). The fluorescein appearance test for lacrimal obstruction. *Annals Ophthalmol.*, 11, 237.

Guzek, J. P., Ching, A. S., Hoang, T. A. *et al.* (1997). Clinical and radiologic lacrimal testing in patients with epiphora. *Ophthalmology*, 104, 1875–81.

Hurwitz, J. J. (1978). Investigation and treatment of epiphora due to lid laxity. *Trans. Ophthal. Soc. UK*, 98, 69–70.

MacEwen, C. J. and Young, J. D. H. (1991). The fluorescein disappearance test (FDT): an evaluation of its use in infants. *J. Paed. Ophthal. Strab.*, 28, 302–5.

Malhotra, R. and Olver, J. M. (2000). Diagrammatic representation of lacrimal disease. *Eye*, 14, 358–63.

Tucker, N. A. and Codere, F. (1994). The effect of fluorescein volume on lacrimal outflow transit time. *Ophth. Plastic Reconstr. Surg.*, 10, 256–9.

Welham, R. A. N. (1998). Investigations for patients undergoing lacrimal surgery. *Eye*, 12, 334–6.

Zappia, R. J. and Milder, B. (1972a). Lacrimal drainage function. I. The Jones fluorescein test. *Am. J. Ophthalmol.*, 74, 154–9.

Zappia, R. J. and Milder, B. (1972b). Lacrimal drainage function. II. The fluorescein dye disappearance test. *Am. J. Ophthalmol.*, 74, 160–2.

Nasal examination:

Enzer, Y. R. and Shorr, N. (1997). The Jones IE test: cobalt blue endoscopic primary dye test of lacrimal excretory function. *Ophthal. Plast. Reconstr. Surg.*, 13, 204.

Olver, J. M. and Minasian, M. (1998). Nasal endoscopy for ophthalmologists. *CME J. Ophthalmol.*, 2, 73–7.

Radiology:

Francis, I. C., Kappagoda, M. B., Cole, I. E. *et al.* (1999). Computer tomography of the lacrimal drainage system: retrospective study of 107 cases of dacryostenosis. *Ophthal. Plast. Reconstr. Surg.*, 15, 217–26.

Galloway, J. E., Kavic, T. A. and Raflo, G. T. (1984). Digital subtraction macrodacryocystography. *Ophthalmology*, 91, 956–62.

Hanna, I. T., MacEwen, C. J. and Kennedy, N. (1992). Lacrimal scintillography in the diagnosis of epiphora. *Nuclear Med. Comm.*, 13, 416–20.

Hurwitz, J. J., Maisey, M. N. and Welham, R. A. N. (1975). Quantitative lacrimal scintillography. *Br. J. Ophthalmol.*, 59, 308–12.

Jedrzynski, M. S. and Bullock, J. D. (1998). Radionuclide dacryocystography. *Orbit*, 17, 1–25.

Kallman, J. E., Foster, J. A., Wulc, A. E. *et al.* (1997). Computer tomography in lacrimal outflow obstruction. *Ophthalmology*, 104, 676–82.

Lloyd, G. A. G. and Welham, R. A. N. (1972) Subtraction macrodacryocystography. *Br. J. Radiol.*, 47, 379–82.

Lloyd, G. A. S., Jones, B. R. and Welham, R. A. N. (1972). Intubation macrodacryocystography. *Br. J. Ophthalmol.*, 56, 600–3.

Mannor, G. E. and Millman, A. L. (1992). The prognostic value of pre-operative dacryocystography in endoscopic intranasal dacryocystorhinostomy. *Am. J. Ophthalmol.*, 113, 134–7.

Massoud, T. F., Whittet, H. B. and Anslow, P. (1993). CT-dacryocystography for nasolacrimal duct obstruction following paranasal sinus surgery. *Br. J. Radiol.*, 66, 223–7.

Wearne, M. J., Pitts, J., Frank, J. and Rose, G. E. (1999). Comparison of dacryocystography aand lacrimal scintigraphy in the diagnosis of functional nasolacrimal duct obstruction. *Br. J. Ophthalmol.*, 83, 1032–5.

CHAPTER 4

Paediatric Lacrimal Surgery

In this chapter the embryology and lacrimal system variations are outlined, the management of congenital nasolacrimal duct obstruction is described and the indications for paediatric DCR are summarized.

Embryology

1. *Embryonic lacrimal plate.* In the 10–12 mm embryo, a strand or cord of thickened epithelium (surface ectoderm) forms in the rudimentary naso-optic fissure.
2. *Solid lacrimal cord.* In the 13–14 mm embryo, this solid cord of epithelial cells grows down into the mesenchyme, detaches from the surface and becomes encompassed by mesenchymal cells. At this stage, the lacrimal cord has no connection to the nasal mucosa or eyelid borders.
3. *Lacrimal cord grows.* In the 14–16 mm embryo, the epithelial cord grows towards the eyelid (cephalic) and towards the nasal cavity. The canalicular buds and early sac remain solid for a while (Figure 4.1).

4. *Canalization.* In the 38–40 mm embryo, around 12 weeks' gestation, the lumina of several segments are established, starting at the ocular end of the cord. The horizontal canaliculi establish a lumen before the vertical sac and duct. Canalization of the sac and nasolacrimal duct proceeds slowly in an infero-medial direction during months 4 and 5 (Figure 4.2).
5. *Punctal development.* The eyelids separate at around 5 months' gestation, at which time the puncta open.
6. *Final canalization of the lower end of the nasolacrimal duct.* The point of coalescence between the nasal end of the cord and the mucosa of the inferior nasal meatus is the last portion to become patent. The lacrimal nasal membrane (valve of Hasner), ruptures at some point between 6 months' gestation to beyond term.

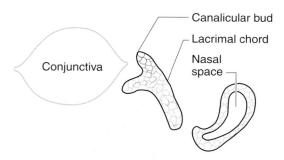

Figure 4.1

Embryological budding of lacrimal cord (based on a drawing by Duke-Elder, 1963).

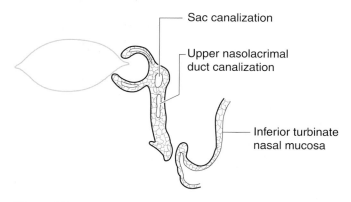

Figure 4.2

Embryological canalization of lacrimal cord (based on a drawing by Duke-Elder, 1963).

Lacrimal system variations

Congenital atresia

The cord of epithelial cells may remain solid at various places.

1. *Punctal atresia.* Failure of the conjunctiva overlying the canaliculus to dehisce when the eyelids open. A membrane persists.
2. *Absent canaliculus.* Failure of a lacrimal budding or canalization.
3. *Duplicated canaliculus and fistula.* Multiple buds sprout towards one or other eyelid or the skin.
4. *Lacrimal sac fistula.* Additional budding from the sac to the skin is a likely cause. It is epithelial lined.
5. *Nasolacrimal duct diverticulae.* Additional sprouting from the side of the nasolacrimal duct.
6. *Nasolacrimal duct lower atresia.* Failure of canalization of the lower end in congenital nasolacrimal duct obstruction. There is a persistent membrane formed by two layers of cells from the lining of the nasolacrimal duct and from the nasal mucosa.
7. *Anomalies from facial clefts.* Parts of the lacrimal system can be missing or obstructed in the clefting syndromes, e.g. Goldenhar's syndrome and amniotic band syndrome. Severe clefting will leave a broad part of the canaliculi and sac missing.

The nasolacrimal ostium in the inferior meatus

This opening into the inferior meatus is very variable in its anatomy, with two distinct types recognized:

1. *Apical.* The ostium lies at the highest point of the inferior nasal meatus, and is permanently open and wide-mouthed without an obvious mucosal flap or valve of Hasner.
2. *Lateral wall.* The ostium is located in an oblique groove on the lateral wall of the inferior nasal meatus, is slit-like and guarded by a mucosal valve of Hasner.

Whether apical or lateral wall, the nasolacrimal duct ostium is located at the junction of the anterior and middle thirds of the inferior meatus. In an adult this is approximately 1.5 cm cephalad to the nasal floor; less in children. A normal ostium is visible with an angled rigid endoscope in the inferior meatus, angled upwards.

Congenital nasolacrimal duct obstruction

Congenital nasolacrimal duct obstruction (CNLDO) is the commonest cause of childhood epiphora. Other causes include the congenital atresias (punctum, canaliculus etc.), craniofacial disorders, and other pathology in an older child (Figure 4.3).

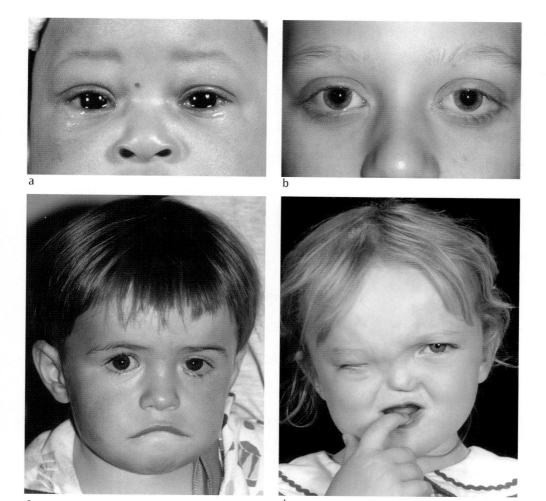

Figure 4.3

a) Infant with bilateral epiphora from congenital nasolacrimal duct obstruction.
b) Five-year-old with bilateral (left more than right) epiphora from chronic mucosal swelling secondary to severe hayfever. Syringing was patent.
c) Two-year-old with left persistent epiphora and mattering from congenital nasolacrimal duct obstruction.
d) Three-year-old with craniofacial disorder consisting of right microphthalmos, heminasal atrophy with absent nasolacrimal duct and cleft through proximal lacrimal system. She has a lacrimal sac mucocoele.

Cause of CNLDO

Failure of initial opening of nasolacrimal duct into the inferior meatus by birth, at the level of the valve of Hasner, or stenosis of the opening from narrowed nasolacrimal duct or hypertrophied inferior turbinate. It represents a delay in the maturation of the lacrimal system and nose (Figure 4.4).

Practice point: The inferior turbinate can be obstructing the opening of the nasolacrimal duct, resulting in functional epiphora. This is still regarded as part of congenital nasolacrimal duct obstruction, as it causes the same symptoms, but may persist longer.

Incidence of CNLDO

At birth, up to 50 per cent of nasolacrimal ducts are still not patent. Spontaneous perforation occurs rapidly in the first 3–4 weeks, and therefore only a few infants have symptomatic epiphora and/or stickiness shortly after birth (1.25–20 per cent).

Symptoms

The onset of symptoms occurs during the first to third weeks after birth, with a few commencing at any time up to 3–5 months. Unilateral > bilateral.

Symptoms include:

1. Epiphora and mattering, unilateral > bilateral – commonest symptoms
2. Mucous discharge from mucocoele
3. Peri-ocular skin soreness and excoriation
4. Acute/chronic dacryocystitis
   - Onset 1–6 weeks with acute congenital dacryocoele
   - Onset 18–24 months.

Practice point: True conjunctivitis is rare. Usually the mother mistakes chronic mattering from dried tears, or mucus expressed from sac, for infection.

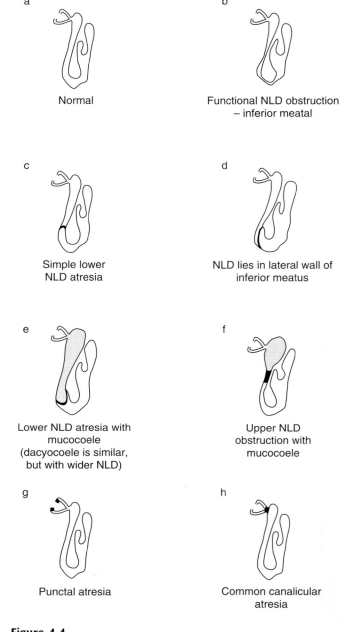

a   Normal

b   Functional NLD obstruction – inferior meatal

c   Simple lower NLD atresia

d   NLD lies in lateral wall of inferior meatus

e   Lower NLD atresia with mucocoele (dacyocoele is similar, but with wider NLD)

f   Upper NLD obstruction with mucocoele

g   Punctal atresia

h   Common canalicular atresia

Figure 4.4

Diagrams showing range of lacrimal system findings in the newborn.

Natural history

Spontaneous resolution is very rapid during the first month of life, 96 per cent resolve in the first year without intervention, and a further 60 per cent resolve in the second year of life. Further resolution continues slowly after that – there will still be some children aged 2–5 years whose symptoms will resolve spontaneously, especially if there is functional obstruction (Table 4.1).

Table 4.1 Probability of resolution of epiphora from CNLDO by age 1 year (derived from MacEwan and Young, 1991). NB: Further resolution may occur in subsequent years

Child's age (months)	Chance of resolution (%)
1	96
3	90
6	75
8	49
10	23
11	5
12	0

Outpatients examination

Exclude absent puncta or accessory canaliculi, identify mucocoele, dacryocoele, and craniofacial disorder. Identify the high tear meniscus and do the dye disappearance test using a blue light. Dacryocystography (under general anaesthesia) is not recommended. Dacryoscintigraphy may be informative, but is usually not required.

Management

Non-surgical management (conservative treatment)

1. Avoid topical antibiotics unless there is conjunctival injection
2. Wipe sticky lids and lashes with cold boiled water
3. Apply paraffin ointment to sore periocular skin
4. Perform lacrimal sac massage.

Educate the parents by informing them of the natural history of the epiphora and avoidance of frequent and unnecessary topical antibiotics. Simple lid bathing and paraffin ointment helps the appearance – often the parent is very embarrassed by the child's epiphora and stickiness, and crèche staff are concerned that there is an infection.

The parent can massage the area of the sac below the medial canthal tendon with a little finger (nail cut short!); this increases the hydrostatic pressure in the lacrimal system and helps express the fluid/mucus into the conjunctival fornix. Massage may accelerate opening of the lower end of the nasolacrimal duct.

Probing

When to probe

Young *et al.* (1997), in a controlled prospective study, showed that probing and syringing the nasolacrimal duct at age 12–14 months was effective compared with spontaneous resolution at 15 months. However, by 24 months there was no statistical difference between the two groups.

Wait until at least 10–12 months before probing unless there is a congenital dacryocoele or acute dacryocystitis, in which case early neonatal probing is the treatment of choice after medical treatment. There is no harm in waiting until 18–24 months before probing, if this is the parents' preference.

Some authors have suggested higher success rates from early probing, but this is likely to include many children with spontaneous resolution. There is no clear-cut evidence that early probing is beneficial.

Practice point: Many parents are reluctant for their child to have a procedure under anaesthesia. In mild cases of epiphora from CNLDO, waiting until the child is aged 18 months before probing is reasonable.

The effectiveness of probing reduces with age because more severe obstructions remain after the initial high rates of spontaneous opening of a simple membrane, and it is more likely that intubation or DCR will be required (Table 4.2).

Table 4.2 Effectiveness of probing (primary and subsequent), from a retrospective study by Mannor *et al.*, 1999

Age probed (years)	Percentage resolution
1	92
2	89
3	80
4	71
5	42

How to do a simple syringe and probing (lacrimal examination under anaesthetic)

1. General anaesthesia with a laryngeal mask is preferred.
2. Examine the eyelids and puncta, exclude fistula/accessory canaliculus, exclude mucocoele by pressing over the lacrimal sac.
3. Syringe and probing equipment:
   - Disposable 26 g lacrimal cannula on a 2 ml syringe with saline/diluted fluorescein
   - Nettleship punctum dilator
   - Set of double-ended Bowman probes – use the size 00:0, or 1:2 in an older child.
4. Dilate the punctum. Insert the Nettleship dilator vertically into the lower or upper punctum, then, with the eyelid on stretch, horizontally dilate the proximal canaliculus.
5. First syringing. Insert the lacrimal canula into the mid-canaliculus and irrigate approximately 1 ml. If there is reflux, identify via which canaliculus is affected. Advance gently into the sac and irrigate – mucus may regurgitate. NB: Check the patency of the other canaliculus. Then proceed to gentle probing.

TIP

Lateral traction on the eyelid straightens the canaliculus and prevents kinking it with the lacrimal canula. Avoid the risk of proximal false passage when syringing and probing.

6. Probe the nasolacrimal duct. Introduce the size 00 Bowman probe into the canaliculus as far as the firm stop of the medial sac wall; withdraw minimally into the sac lumen, and at the same time swing the probe vertically down the nasolacrimal duct. The probe should lie flat on the child's brow, directed slightly posteriorly down the duct. This manoeuvre should be done gently, without pressure (Figure 4.5).

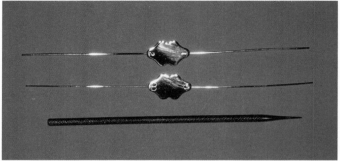

a

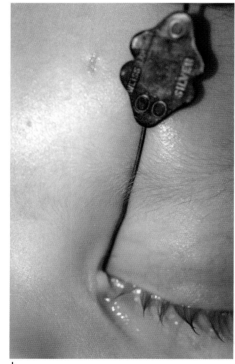

b

Figure 4.5

a) Probing set with Nettleship dilator and smaller-sized Bowman probes.

b) Bowman probe (size 00) passed horizontally along lower canaliculus with eyelid on stretch, then swung vertically down nasolacrimal duct. The external part lies on the child's eyebrow.

TIP

Each end of the Bowman probe measures 5 cm; therefore by measuring the length of exterior probe before the finger hold, you can calculate the distance reached down the duct or into the nose.

7. Perforate the membrane and enter the nose. A 'pop' should be felt as the probe is passed through the membrane at the lower end of the nasolacrimal duct (valve of Hasner), then a firmness as the probe settles on the nasal floor. There should be minimal or no bleeding from the punctum and nose. Confirm patency by direct endonasal viewing of the probe in the inferior meatus (see below, endoscopic endonasal monitoring). It is not recommended to stick a second metal object along the floor blindly for metal on metal touch, as this can traumatize the nasal mucosa and is often inaccurate.

TIP

If it is an easy probe with the size 00, it is not necessary to repeat with the 0 size. Each time a probe is passed, the risk of mucosal damage and false passage increases. If the passage of the probe felt a bit tight at the lower end of the nasolacrimal duct, gently repeat with a size 0 or even 1 in an older child aged 2+ years. Avoid a size 2 probe, as this risks canalicular damage.

8. Second syringing. After probing, repeat the syringing with 1–2 ml saline and fluorescein and confirm patency by looking in the nose with an endoscope or aspirating fluorescein-stained fluid from the throat with a small soft suction tube.

TIP

If a nasal endoscope is not available to view the fluorescein–saline emerging into the inferior meatus, an apparent negative second syringing with some regurgitation does not always indicate a failed probing. Do not go back and repeat the probing.

Post-operatively, topical steroid-antibiotics are instilled for between 1 and 3 weeks, depending on the severity of the CNLDO. The patient is reviewed in clinic in 6 weeks.

Complications

Complications per-probing include:

1. Bleeding
2. Inability to pass the probe down the nasolacrimal duct
3. Inability to confirm patency on second syringing
4. Suspicion or confirmation of false passage
5. The probe remains submucosal in the lateral wall and touches bony maxilla, but not within the nose.

Complications post-probing include:

1. The above complications with persistence of symptoms
2. The probe appearing to be easily passed, but the symptoms persist
3. A confirmed successful probing and syringing, but symptoms persist
4. Acute dacryocystitis and preseptal orbital cellulitis, especially if a false passage is made.

Syringe and probing with balloon catheter dilation

A 3 mm diameter balloon is passed into the nasolacrimal duct transcanalicular and used to dilate the opening of the duct into the inferior meatus at the valve of Hasner. For details of the technique, see Chapter 8. This technique is usually reserved for repeat probing, and may include silicone intubation.

Congenital dacryocoele or congenital lacrimal sac mucocoele

The exception to probing and syringing at age 1 year is congenital dacryocoele, where early probing at less than 6 weeks of age may be indicated.

Congenital dacryocoele is an uncommon neonatal swelling of the lacrimal sac. It is typically a tense, bluish swelling present at birth or within 1–4 weeks. Approximately 25 per cent have bilateral dacryocoeles. Other terms used in the past include congenital nasolacrimal sac mucocoele, dacryocystocele, amniotocele or amniocele, neonatal mucocoele, and acute neonatal dacryocystitis.

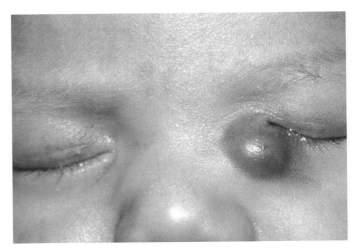

Figure 4.6

Inflamed left congenital dacryocoele in neonate (3 weeks old). There is a tense acute dacryocystitis.

Congenital dacryocoele can become red and inflamed with an acute dacryocystitis and the child febrile and ill. Recognize a spectrum of this condition from the quiet bluish dacryocoele to the red infected dacryocoele, as the management depends on the severity (Figure 4.6).

There is both a functional block above the sac and atresia at the lower end of the nasolacrimal duct. Recognize that the entire sac and nasolacrimal duct are expanded (Figure 4.7). There is an inferior mucocoele extending intranasally in approximately 75 per cent of cases. The inferior mucocoele may extend just into the inferior meatus or further into the nasal space, where it causes respiratory distress, especially if bilateral (Figure 4.8). Nasal endoscopic examination will reveal the extent of the intranasal cyst extension and assist internal drainage and marsupialization (Figure 4.9).

Differential diagnosis of congenital dacryocoele:
- Meningoencephalocoele
- Orbital cellulites
- Rhabdomyosarcoma
- Capillary haemangioma
- Dermoid cyst.

Investigations

When the diagnosis remains uncertain MRI or CT scanning is helpful, but is not indicated routinely (see Figure 4.7).

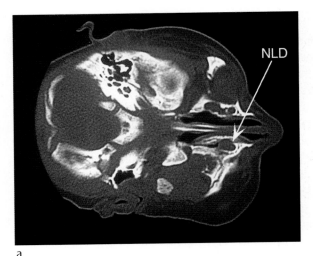

a

b

Figure 4.7

Congenital dacryocoele in 3-week-old neonate.
a) MRI showing widened nasolacrimal duct on affected side.
b) CT showing very enlarged lacrimal sac.

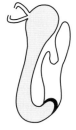

Lower NLD atresia with dacryocoele and large inferior mucocoele

Figure 4.8

Diagram showing widened nasolacrimal duct with inferior mucocoele forming an intranasal cyst.

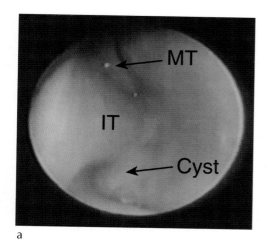

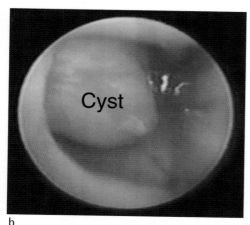

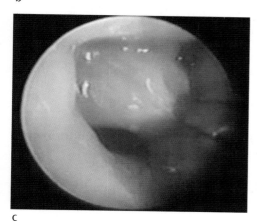

Figure 4.9

a) Right endoscopic view of intranasal cyst in a 17-day-old child with congenital dacryocoele. MT = middle turbinate, IT = inferior turbinate. The pale cyst fills the right inferior meatus.

b) Close up of cyst in inferior meatus. NVR blade is then used to incise the cyst – mucous will drain intranasally.

c) The deflated cyst wall must now be removed with forceps to marsupialize the opening.

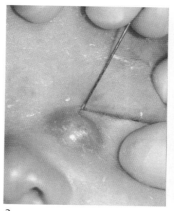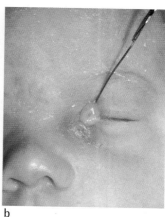

Figure 4.10

Left congenital dacryocoele.
a) The left inflamed dacryocoele and nasolacrimal duct is probed via the lower canaliculus.
b) Pressure over the sac with the probe *in situ* causes expression of mucus and pus proximally. The probe is lying on the nasal floor, but has been ineffective in draining the inferior mucocoele. High pressure syringing with fluorescein–saline is then used to blow out the inferior mucocoele.

Management

1. Quiet dacryocoele (neonatal mucocoele): massage, warm compresses.
2. Inflamed dacryocoele (acute neonatal dacryocystitis): intravenous antibiotics for 5–7 days. Examination under anaesthetic with probing, syringing and nasal endoscopy. Do *not* drain the abscess via the skin as in adult acute dacryocystitis, but drain internally into the nose. The mucosa over the inferior mucocoele (intranasal cyst) is incised and marsupialized by transcanalicular syringing with saline to cause 'blow-out', or transnasal surgical/laser excision/ablation may be used. Up to 7 ml of mucus/pus is contained within the enlarged sac, nasolacrimal duct and inferior mucocoele (see Figures 4.9, 4.10).

Endoscopic endonasal monitoring of syringe and probing

A rigid endoscope is placed in the inferior meatus to monitor correct placement of the probe and effective

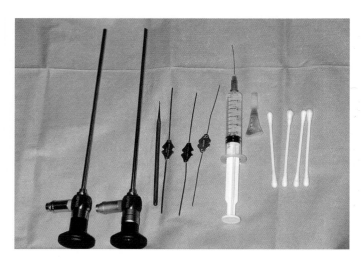

Figure 4.11

Left to right: Hopkins 0° or 30° rigid endoscope, 2.7 mm, 3 mm or 4 mm diameter; Nettleship dilator and Bowman probes; disposable lacrimal cannula 26 g on 2 ml syringe with fluorescein–saline; cotton buds for applying adrenaline 1 in 1000 onto inferior meatus mucosa.

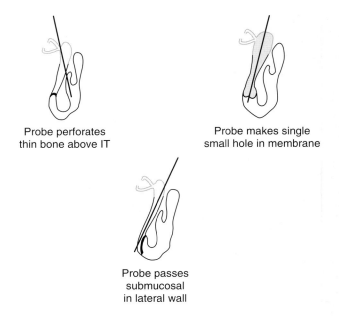

Figure 4.12

Diagrams showing the potential problems with unmonitored probing.

syringing. If endoscopic monitoring is not available, the simple syringe and probing should be restricted to primary probing only.

Equipment

In addition to the equipment shown in Figure 4.11, a Freer's elevator is required to infracture or push the inferior turbinate medially. A fine sucker is useful to hold the inferior turbinate displaced medially and to aspirate the mucus drained into the inferior meatus.

Indications

Congenital nasolacrimal duct obstruction with or without mucocoele or dacryocystitis.

1. If possible, primary syringe and probing.
2. If possible, marsupialization of inferior mucocoele in congenital dacryocoele (use 2.7 or 3 mm diameter because neonate).
3. Endoscopic monitoring of secondary syringe and probing.
4. Lacrimal system intubation.

Why perform endoscopic endonasal monitoring of syringe and probing?

The problem with simple syringe and probing is that the probe can be in the wrong place or ineffective (Figure 4.12).

Endoscopic endonasal monitoring helps to rectify these problems.

How to perform endoscopic endonasal monitoring of syringe and probing

In addition to the standard examination under anaesthetic, the nasal mucosa is decongested and nasal endoscopy is done whilst irrigating and probing. If necessary, the membrane over the lower end of the nasolacrimal duct is cut down (marsupialized) to improve drainage.

1. The endoscope is placed in the nasal space and the floor and inferior turbinate identified.
2. The Freer elevator is used to push the anterior part of the inferior turbinate medially for a good view of

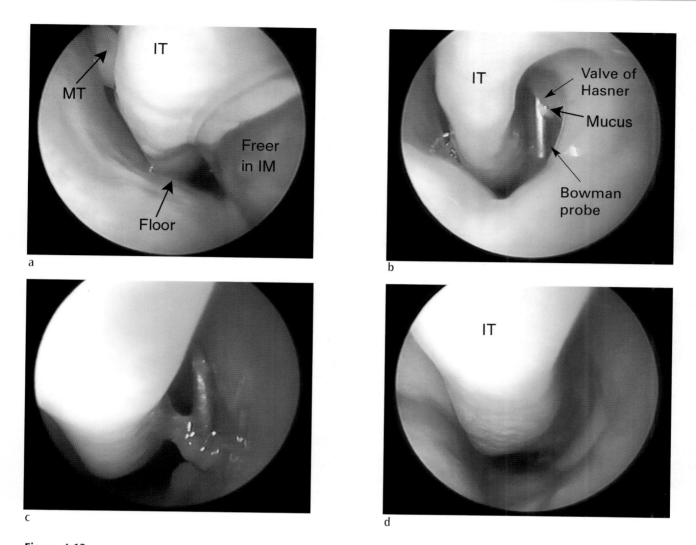

Figure 4.13

Epiphora from simple lower nasolacrimal duct atresia. Left nasal space viewed with 4 mm 30° rigid endoscope. IT = inferior turbinate, IM = inferior meatus.
a) Freer elevator displacing inferior turbinate medial.
b) Probe visible in meatus with mucous plug drainage.
c) Higher magnification of more mucus.
d) Fluorescein–saline irrigation. Note that the opening lies in a groove in the upper part of the inferior meatus lateral wall. There is a slight mucosal bulge anterior and superior to the groove, which is of normal appearance.

the roof and lateral wall of the inferior meatus.

3. After initial syringing confirms obstruction, the probe is inserted. If it is seen sliding down the lateral wall underneath the mucosa, it is withdrawn slightly and the direction altered to make it emerge into the meatus.

4. Pressing on the lacrimal sac to increase the hydrostatic pressure helps drain a plug of mucus or a rush of mucus.

5. The probe is withdrawn and a second fluorescein-saline irrigation done to wash away backed-up mucus and to confirm patency (Figure 4.13).

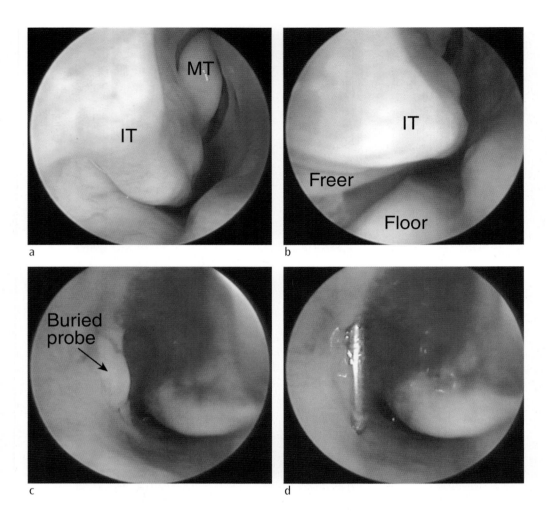

Figure 4.14

Three-year-old who had persistent epiphora following simple probing.
a) Right nasal space. MT = middle turbinate, IT = inferior turbinate.
b) Freer elevator used to gain access to inferior meatus. IT = inferior turbinate.
c) Right inferior meatus. The probe has been passed and come to a firm stop on the floor. It has remained in the lateral nasal wall, submucosally.
d) The probe is repositioned and now emerges into the apex of the inferior meatus.

Failed probing

Simple syringe and probing is generally effective, but a few fail, especially in the older child where there is persistence of more severe CNLDO or pathology caused by the previous probing.

Why simple probing may fail:
1. Probe is unable to pierce membrane, or hole made is inadequate for drainage
2. Probe remains in submucosal space on lateral wall meatus
3. Probe makes false passage
4. Probe has damaged canalicular or nasolacrimal duct mucosa
5. Probing appeared successful and syringed patent, but there is functional epiphora
6. Initial pathology was more extensive than simple lower nasolacrimal duct atresia, e.g. mid- or high nasolacrimal duct block.

What to do if probing fails and epiphora persists or recurs

If simple syringe and probing has failed and the symptoms are still present or recur (usually within 6 weeks), list the patient for examination under anaesthetic with endoscopic endonasal monitoring of syringe and probing.

Wait 3 months before this second probing unless there is dacryocystitis, where early intervention is recommended. If the repeat probing is easy and the cause is probably that the probe remained initially submucosal, you may avoid intubation (Figure 4.14).

If endoscopic endonasal monitoring of syringe and probing fails, repeat, with silicone intubation. Only consider dacryocystorhinostomy if intubation is unlikely to succeed, for instance, in an extensive block where the probe cannot pass beyond the sac.

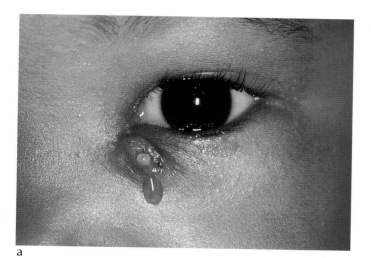

Figure 4.15

Left acute dacryocystitis with spontaneous percutaneous drainage in a 2-year-old boy, unresponsive to topical and systemic antibiotics.
a) Before probing.
b) Left inferior meatus. Probe emerging through valve of Hasner. IT = inferior turbinate.
c) Copious intranasal mucus drainage.
The child made a full recovery.

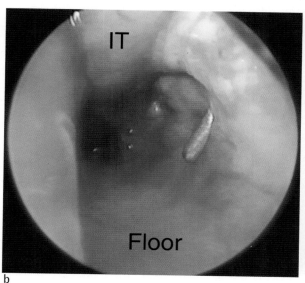

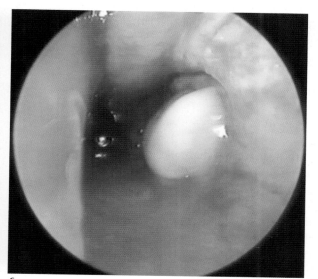

Acute dacryocystitis in children

Endoscopic endonasal monitoring of probing is the initial treatment of choice, to enable intranasal drainage of mucus/pus. The decision whether to insert tubes is made at the time of probing, and depends on the degree of nasolacrimal block felt and the amount of inferior mucosal damage/inflammation encountered (Figure 4.15).

Congenital functional epiphora

There is persistent epiphora in the presence of normal syringe and probing. Either the lower end of the nasolacrimal duct is stenotic, or the ostium is partially blocked by a hypertrophied or laterally inclined inferior turbinate.

Management

1. Wait. The lacrimal system and nose may mature and achieve spontaneous resolution.

2. Endoscopic endonasal monitoring of syringe and probing to confirm, then intubation for 3 months.

Bicanalicular silicone intubation

Indications

The indications for temporary placement of silicone tubes include:

1. Failed endoscopic endonasal monitored syringe and probing
2. Persistent functional epiphora
3. Clinical judgement – mucosal opening inflamed or more than simple lower nasolacrimal duct atresia, for instance an obvious focal nasolacrimal block that can be overcome.

Different tubing

There are two main types of silicone tubing commonly used:

1. Crawford tubes – external diameter 0.6 mm. The silicone tubing is attached to two flexible metallic bodkins, and the retrieval device is a hook (Figure 4.16).
2. Ritleng tubes, external diameter 0.64 mm. The same hook can be used, or a small forceps. Instead of bodkins, the Ritleng tubes are passed down the centre of an introducing probe (Figure 4.17).

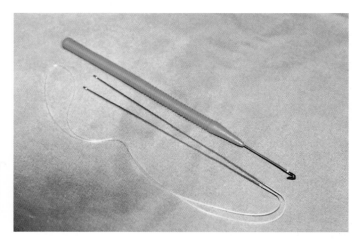

Figure 4.16

Crawford-type silicone intubation set with retrieval hook. The bodkins are quite flexible.

How to insert Crawford tubes

Insertion is under general anaesthetic and with nasal mucosal decongestion.

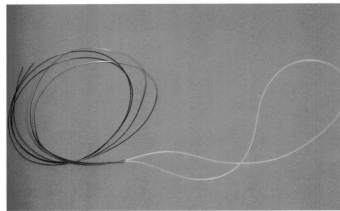

a

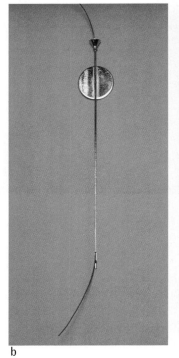 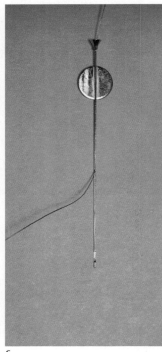

b   c

Figure 4.17

a) Ritleng intubation consists of a central length of silicone and graded blue polypropylene introducing ends.
b) The polypropylene is threaded through the stainless steel Ritleng introducer.
c) The introducer has a groove all along one side, through which the thinnest (light blue) part of the introducing ends can be removed.

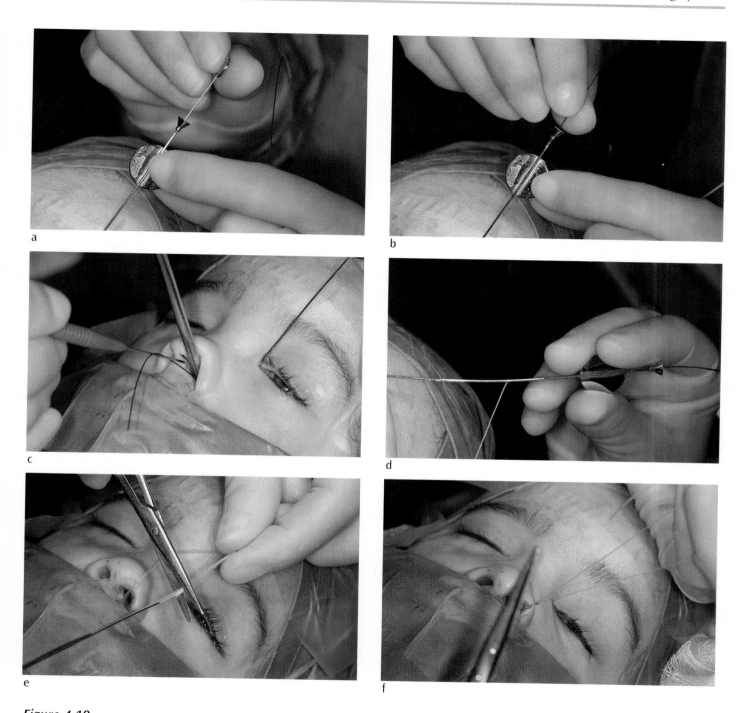

Figure 4.18

Left Ritleng intubation.
a) Introducer inserted into lacrimal system and stillette removed.
b) Prolene introducing end threaded down introducer until seen in nose in inferior meatus.
c) Crawford hook retrieval of blue polypropylene end under external monitoring.
d) Introducer removed before prolene is pulled out of the nostril and prolene slipped out of side groove.
e) Prolene ends trimmed.
f) Silicone knotted – knot remains in inferior meatus.

After punctal dilation the metal bodkins are introduced as for probing, one via the upper and one via the lower canaliculus. Each bodkin is observed and retrieved from the inferior meatus using the hook, under direct endoscopic view. The bodkins are cut off and the tubes tied together, checking the tension and location of the knot in the inferior meatus.

How to insert Ritleng tubes

General anaesthesia and nasal preparation is similar to that for Crawford tubes.

1. Dilate lower and upper puncta
2. Probe the lacrimal system to confirm route
3. Infracture the inferior turbinate to see the inferior meatus well
4. Insert Ritleng introducer with stillette via one canaliculus, into the sac and down the nasolacrimal duct into the inferior meatus; remove stillette
5. Feed polypropylene down centre of the introducer until seen in the inferior meatus
6. Using the retrieval device or forceps, pull the introducing end out towards the nostril and hold it
7. Remove the introducer and slip the tubing out of its vertical groove
8. Pull the introducing ends fully out of the nostril and repeat with the other canaliculus and end
9. Cut the polypropylene ends off and tie the silicone tubing with knots in the inferior meatus as for Crawford tubes, then trim the ends
10. Irrigate the lacrimal system with fluorescein–saline.

See Figure 4.18.

TIP

If using the hook retriever, it is best to have the open groove on the introducer facing posterior, to direct the polypropylene introducing end posteriorly – it is easier to catch in the hook and pull anteriorly. If the retrieval forceps are used, have the groove facing anterior to direct the polypropylene anteriorly towards the forceps.

For precision and to minimize mucosal damage, monitor the intubation endonasally using the rigid endoscope (Figure 4.19).

Removal of tubes

This is best done under a short second general anaesthetic, up to 3 months later. The nose is decongested and the tube's knot identified in the inferior meatus; infracture may be required. Once identified, the tube is cut at the medial canthus and retrieved from the nose. The lacrimal system is then irrigated to wash out any backed up debris and confirm patency.

Potential tube complications

1. Cheesewiring punctum
2. Lateral displacement
3. Scarring in inferior meatus
4. Persistent epiphora.

Punctal agenesis

Many children with single punctal agenesis are asymptomatic, and reach old age before the absent punctum is noted when they develop epiphora from nasolacrimal duct stenosis.

At probing, one or more puncta may appear missing. If an upper punctum is missing, this is unlikely to be the main cause of epiphora and the nasolacrimal duct should be probed to detect coexistent CNLDO.

Practice point: If there is a single punctal agenesis and symptoms, suspect associated nasolacrimal duct obstruction.

Decide if there is simple agenesis or more extensive underlying canalicular agenesis.

Simple agenesis

There is a visible papilla and membrane overlying the summit. Use a fine needle to twirl down through the membrane into a normal ampulla and canaliculus, then probe to confirm a normal nasolacrimal duct. Do not intubate unless there is a nasolacrimal duct indication.

Punctal agenesis with canalicular atresia

If there is no visible papilla or membrane present, suspect underlying canalicular agenesis.

If one punctum is missing, the child may be asymptomatic or have epiphora and/or stickiness or a history of dacryocystitis; therefore probe via the other puncta to detect coexistent CNLDO. If there is severe

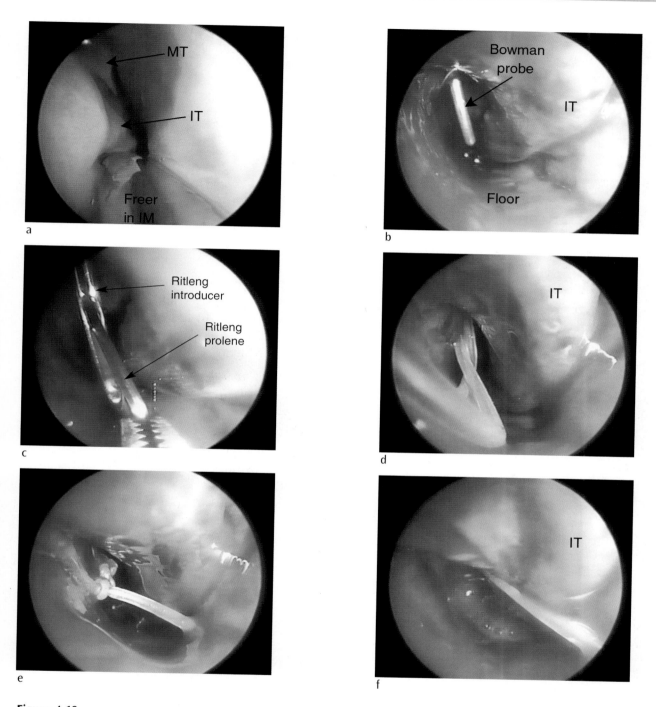

Figure 4.19

Endonasal monitoring of right Ritleng intubation in 2-year-old.
a) Freer elevator infractures/displaces medially the anterior part of the inferior turbinate. MT = middle turbinate, IT = inferior turbinate, IM = inferior meatus.
b) Bowman probe through valve of Hasner in middle meatus. IT = inferior turbinate.
c) Ritleng introducer and polypropylene introducing end visible on nasal floor. Ritleng forceps used to grab prolene end.
d) Silicone tubes both through.
e) Silicone knots in inferior meatus.
f) Positive endoscopic dye test on syringing (silicone pulled on stretch to demonstrate).

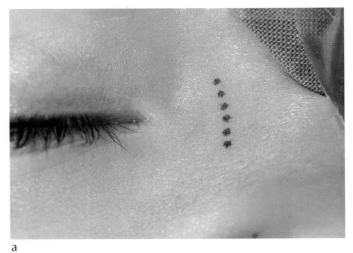

a

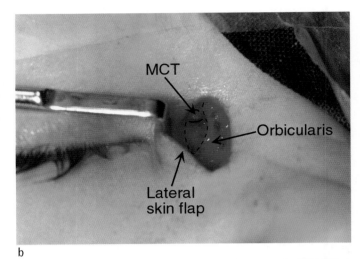

b

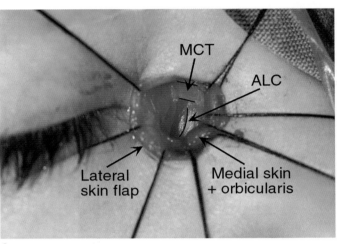

c

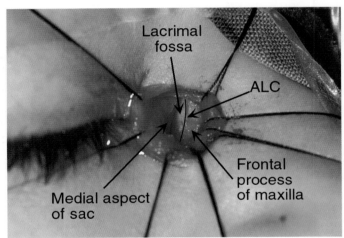

d

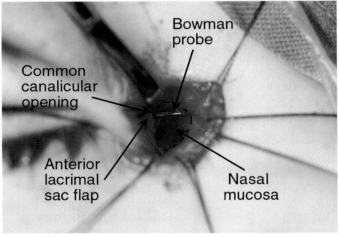

e

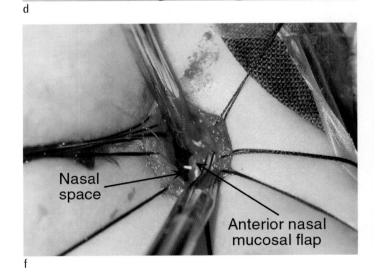

f

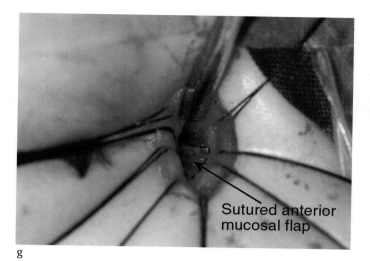

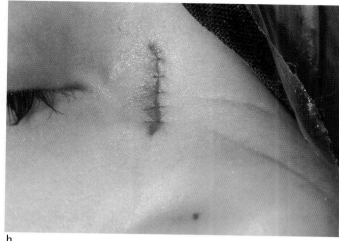

g

h

Figure 4.20

Right DCR in 2½-year-old.
a)   Straight skin incision approximately 10 mm long, 10 mm from medial canthal angle.
b)   Fison retractor holding lateral skin flap. MCT = medial canthal tendon.
c)   Traction sutures in place. Anterior lacrimal crest (ALC), frontal process of maxilla and lacrimal fossa identified.
d)   MCT divided to increase access to medial aspect of sac.
e)   The osteotomy has been done. The sac is opened and Bowman probe passes easily through the common canalicular internal opening.
f)   The nasal mucosal flaps have been cut and the anterior flap is being sutured to the anterior lacrimal sac flap.
g)   The anterior flap is sutured.
h)   The skin is closed with fine absorbable suture.

nasolacrimal duct obstruction, DCR with retrograde intubation or monocanalicular intubation is indicated.

If both the upper and lower puncta are absent and no papilla is found, the epiphora may be mild with no symptoms of stickiness or dacryocystitis. Surgery for this group is difficult, and the alternative is to do nothing. Treatment is external DCR with retrograde intubation via the common canalicular internal opening, if identified. If this is not present, the child will require a Jones bypass tube. If the epiphora is mild, many surgeons recommend waiting until the child is older (e.g. 14–18 years) before considering a Jones tube, as by then the child can make a responsible informed decision.

Practice point: Observation is always an option for punctal and canalicular agenesis.

Dacryocystorhinostomy (DCR) in children

Indications

1.   Unresolved CNLDO after probing or intubation
2.   Punctal agenesis with canalicular atresia
3.   Canalicular atresia
4.   Acquired canalicular disease.

Unresolved CNLDO, i.e. where there is more extensive nasolacrimal duct disease unresponsive to endoscopic endonasal syringe and probing and intubation, responds well to standard external approach DCR (90–93 per cent success rate) or to endonasal DCR. It is better to wait until the child is aged 2–4 years, although DCR performed on younger children aged 12–18 months has not been associated with disturbed bone growth, despite that obvious concern.

Technique for external DCR

See Figure 4.20.
1. Make a short lateral side of nose skin flap incision, and identify medial canthal tendon.
2. Use 6.0 black silk traction sutures, and divide the orbicularis at the anterior lacrimal crest; open the periosteum and expose the lacrimal fossa and the medial wall of the sac.
3. Insert a Bowman probe via the lower or upper canaliculus into the sac, and cut down vertically on the overlying sac mucosa with upper and lower horizontal relieving incisions to create anterior and posterior lacrimal sac mucosal flaps.
4. Perform an osteotomy as in the adult. The ethmoids are not usually prominent in a child.
5. Make a vertical cut down on the nasal mucosa with upper and lower horizontal relieving incisions to create anterior and posterior nasal mucosal flaps.
6. If possible, suture the posterior lacrimal and nasal flaps together with 7.0 Vicryl then the anterior lacrimal and nasal flaps with 7.0 or 6.0 Vicryl. Anterior sutured flaps are adequate.
7. Reposition the orbicularis and skin flap and suture the skin with fine 7.0 or 8.0 Vicryl interrupted sutures, which will dissolve.

For the techniques of DCR with retrograde intubation, canaliculo-DCR and conjunctival-DCR, see Chapter 6.

Congenital lacrimal fistulae

1. Congenital lacrimal fistulae are epithelial lined.
2. They link to the common canaliculus (an accessory canaliculus), lacrimal sac or nasolacrimal duct.
3. Rarely, they are blind ending.
4. They are situated near the medial canthus, or inferonasal to the medial canthal angle.
5. They are often asymptomatic and go undetected for many years, as the canaliculi are often anatomically and functionally normal.
6. No treatment is needed unless there is epiphora.

Management of congenital fistula with epiphora

1. Confirm patent lacrimal system via upper and lower canaliculus.
2. Perform gentle probe of the nasolacrimal duct if CNLDO is suspected.
3. Excise the fistula surgically using a no.11 Barde Parker blade.
4. Further extensive surgery is rarely necessary unless there is a more severe abnormality.

Bibliography

Embryology and anatomy:

Schaeffer, J. P. (1921). The modern conception of the anatomy of the nasolacrimal passageways in man. *Am. J. Ophthalmol.*, 4, 683–5.

Sevel, D. (1981). Development and congenital abnormalities of the nasolacrimal apparatus. *J. Paed. Ophthalmol. Strab.*, 18, 13–19.

Yanagisawa, E. and Yanagisawa, K. (1993). Endoscopic view of ostium of nasolacrimal duct. *Ear Nose Throat J.*, 72, 491–2.

Natural history and probing of congenital nasolacrimal duct obstruction:

Busse, H., Muller, K. M. and Kroll, P. (1980). Radiological and histological findings of the lacrimal passages of newborns. *Arch. Ophthalmol.*, 98, 528–32.

El-Mansoury, J., Calhoun, J. H., Nelson, L. B. and Harley, R. D. (1986). Results of late probing for congenital nasolacrimal duct obstruction. *Ophthalmology*, 93, 1052–4.

Katowitz, J. A. and Welsh, M. G. (1987). Timing of initial probing and irrigation in congenital nasolacrimal duct obstruction. *Ophthalmology*, 94, 698–705.

Kushner, B. J. (1982). Congenital nasolacrimal system obstruction. *Arch. Ophthalmol.*, 100, 597–600.

MacEwan, C. J. and Young, J. D. H. (1991). Epiphora during the first year of life. *Eye*, 5, 596–600.

Mannor, G. E., Rose, G. E., Frimpong-Ansah, K. and Ezra, E. (1999). Factors affecting the success of nasolacrimal duct probing for congenital nasolacrimal duct obstruction. *Am. J. Ophthalmol.*, 127, 616–17.

Paul, T. O. (1985). Medical management of congenital nasolacrimal duct obstruction. *J. Paed. Ophthalmol. Strab.*, 22, 68–70.

Young, J. D. H. and MacEwan, C. J. (1997). Managing congenital lacrimal obstruction in general. *Br. Med. J.*, 315, 293–6.

Young, J. D. H., MacEwan, C. J. and Ogston, S. A. (1996). Congenital nasolacrimal duct obstruction in the second year of life: a multicentre trial of management. *Eye*, 10, 485–91.

Congenital dacryocoele:

Campolattaro, B. N., Lueder, G. T. and Tychsen, L. (1997). Spectrum of paediatric dacryocystitis: medical and surgical management of 54 cases. *J. Paed. Ophthalmol. Strab.*, 34, 143–53.

Divine, R. D., Anderson, R. L. and Bumstead, R. M. (1983). Bilateral congenital lacrimal sac mucocoeles with nasal extension and drainage. *Arch. Ophthalmol.*, 101, 246–8.

Grin, T. R., Mertz, J. S. and Stass-Isern, M. (1991). Congenital nasolacrimal duct cysts in dacryocystocoele. *Ophthalmology*, 98, 1238–42.

Lueder, G. T. (1995). Neonatal dacryocystitis associated with nasolacrimal duct cysts. *J. Paed. Ophthalmol. Strab.*, 32, 102–6.

Lusk, R. P. and Muntz, H. M. (1987). Nasal obstruction in the neonate secondary to nasolacrimal duct cysts. *Int. J. Ped. Otolaryngol.*, 13, 315–22.

Mansour, A. M., Cheng, K. P., Mumma, J. V. *et al.* (1991). Congenital dacryocoele. A collaborative review. *Ophthalmology*, 98, 1744–51.

Paysse, E. A., Coats, D. K., Bernstein, J. M. *et al.* (2000). Management and complications of congenital dacryocele with concurrent intranasal mucocele. *J. AAPOS*, 4, 46–53.

Schnall, B. M. and Christian, C. J. (1996). Conservative treatment of congenital dacryocele. *J. Paed. Ophthalmol. Strab.*, 33, 219–21.

Nasolacrimal duct intubation:

Aggarwal, R. K., Misson, G. P., Donaldson, I. and Willshaw, H. E. (1993). The role of nasolacrimal intubation in the management of childhood epiphora. *Eye*, 7, 760–62.

Punctal agenesis:

Lyons, C. J., Rosser, P. M. and Welham, R. A. N. (1993). The management of punctal agenesis. *Ophthalmology*, 12, 1851–5.

Endonasal endoscopic evaluation of probing:

Ram, B., Barras, C. W., White, P. S. *et al.* (2000). The technique of nasoendoscopy in the evaluation of congenital nasolacrimal duct obstruction in children. *Rhinology*, 38, 83–6.

Balloon catheter dilation:

Becker, B. B., Berry, F. D. and Koller, H. (1996). Balloon catheter dilation for treatment of congenital nasolacrimal duct obstruction. *Am. J. Ophthalmol.*, 121, 304–9.

Paediatric dacryocystorhinostomy:

Doyle, A., Russell, J. and O'Keefe, M. (2000). Paediatric laser dacryocystorhinostomy. *Acta Ophthalmol. Scand.*, 78, 204–5.

Hakin, K. N., Sullivan, T. J., Sharma, A. and Welham, R. A. N. (1994). Paediatric dacryocystorhinostomy. *Aust. NZ J. Ophthalmol.*, 22, 231–5.

Welham, R. A. N. and Hughes, S. M. (1985). Lacrimal surgery in children. *Am. J. Ophthalmol.*, 99, 27–34.

Welham, R. A. N., Bates, A. K. and Stasior, G. O. (1992). Congenital lacrimal fistula. *Eye*, 6, 211–14.

CHAPTER 5

Adult Lacrimal Surgery

In this chapter the management of acute dacryocystitis, epiphora, and discharge from nasolacrimal duct obstruction are described. Dacryocystorhinostomy and post-operative management are covered in depth. For the management of canalicular disease (with or without nasolacrimal duct stenosis), see Chapter 6. For trans-canalicular DCR, see Chapter 8.

The chapter is divided as follows:

Part A: Dacryocystitis

Part B: Dacryocystorhinostomy (DCR)
   I.   External approach
   II. Endonasal endoscopic
       i) Endonasal surgical
       ii) Endonasal laser

Part C: Post-operative management.

Part A: Dacryocystitis

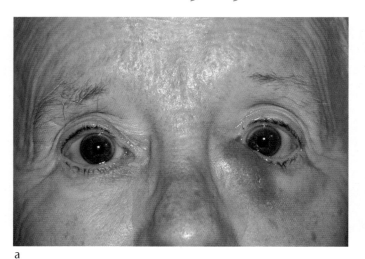

a

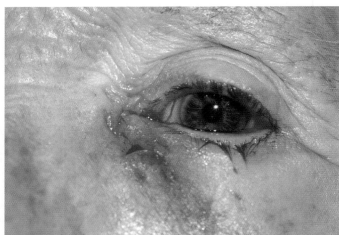

b

Figure 5. 1

a) Left acute dacryocystitis with a palpable abscess.
b) The abscess has been decompressed and all the pus drained. The cruciate incision is visible. The cavity is then packed with ribbon gauze.

Aetiology

Patients with dacryocystitis (Figure 5.1) usually have nasolacrimal duct obstruction (± dacryoliths or lacrimal sac diverticula), and therefore definitive treatment is generally DCR. There are a few cases of acute dacryocystitis where there is normal syringing on resolution and which do not get a recurrence or need DCR. In these cases, the probable cause was a dacryolith, which passed spontaneously down the nasolacrimal duct.

> **Differential diagnosis of acute dacryocystitis:**
> * Acute skin infection
> * Acute ethmoiditis/inflamed ethmoid mucocoele
> * Ruptured dermoid or epidermoid cyst
> * Lacrimal sac tumour.

Dacryocystitis sub-types

1. Sub-acute
2. Acute
3. Chronic.

Sub-acute dacryocystitis

There is a mucocoele with a moderately inflamed wall. Tender and non-reducible on digital pressure, there is a risk of it developing into acute dacryocystitis.

Treatment

Broad spectrum oral antibiotics as indicated. External approach or endonasal DCR with tubes, within 2 months. Leave the tubes in for up to 8 weeks.

Acute dacryocystitis

There is a very painful, enlarged lacrimal sac containing mucus and pus, which cannot escape (non-reducible). The inflamed sac can only expand anteriorly, inferiorly and laterally due to its position in the lacrimal fossa anterior to the orbital septum, and the pus track to the skin surface. When the inflammation spreads beyond the sac wall into the surrounding tissue there may be pericystitis or, if it is more extensive, preseptal orbital cellulitis. It is very rare for acute dacryocystitis to cause a post-septal orbital cellulitis because the sac is anterior to the septum.

The risk of recurrent dacryocystitis is at least 50 per cent in elderly patients if the underlying cause is not addressed – i.e. DCR for nasolacrimal duct obstruction.

Treatment

Initial: Broad-spectrum antibiotics. Palpate the lump to detect the presence of an abscess; if present, do a dacryocystotomy and pack. Some surgeons will do a DCR in the acute phase, bypassing the need for dacryocystotomy.

Later: Most surgeons wait 2–3 weeks (until the inflammation has settled) before proceeding with an external approach DCR and tubes, which allows a membranectomy of the internal common opening to be done if required. Alternatively, do an endonasal DCR and tubes, opening the sac as wide as possible. Leave the tubes in for 8–12 weeks.

Chronic dacryocystitis

Recurrent attacks of acute dacryocystitis lead to chronic dacryocystitis, often with an acquired fistula from the sac to the skin, below the medial canthal tendon.

Treatment

External approach or large surgical endonasal DCR with tubes. An external approach is preferred to exclude lacrimal sac diverticula, biopsy if indicated and excise intra-sac membranes. The fistula will settle without excision (it is not epithelial lined). The common canalicular opening and sac mucosa are quite inflamed; therefore tubes are left in for 12 weeks.

TIP
Wegener's granulomatosis and sarcoidosis cause chronic dacryocystitis, and surgery should include tissue biopsy of the sac and surrounding tissue if these are suspected.

Dacryocystitis: historical perspective

Lacrimal sac abscess (acute dacryocystitis) and resultant lacrimal fistula were treated by sac excision (dacryocystectomy), incision (dacryocystotomy) or cautery from at least the first century BC, with some early records of lacrimal surgery dating back to the time of the Roman and Greek empires.

Dacryocystotomy

Definition: Incision and drainage of abscess in acute dacryocystitis. The abscess cavity is usually packed with ribbon gauze for up to 3 days.

Procedure

This is performed under local anaesthesia: peri-abscess injection of lidocaine with adrenaline.

1. Incise abscess. Use a no. 11 Barde Parker blade to make a large, deep, cruciate skin incision centred over the apex of the abscess.
2. Explore wound and drain abcess. Place the Freer's elevator or closed artery clip deep in the wound, directed towards the lacrimal fossa (postero-medial-inferior), up to a depth of 15–20 mm. An ethmoid mucocoele is excluded by the location of the mass and direction on exploration. Use straight, blunt scissors to open the deep part of the wound, and a free syringe (without needle attached) or sucker to aspirate all the pus.
3. Pack the abscess cavity. Insert ribbon gauze soaked in antibiotic or proflavin deep inside the wound. Leave 2 cm visible out of wound in order to shorten and remove the gauze over the next few days. Apply a light sterile gauze eye pad.
4. Arrange a planned DCR + tubes within 2–4 weeks.

Dacryolithiasis

Lacrimal sac stones (Figure 5.2) are found in up to 15 per cent of DCR operations. Stones consist of dried mucus, lipid and inflammatory cells, and are more likely to be found in chronically inflamed sacs with increased

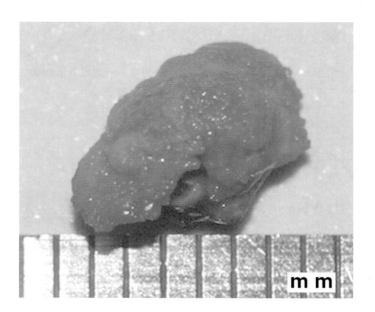

m m

mucin-producing cells, with or without complete nasolacrimal duct obstruction. They can be small soft flakes, multiple small granules or a large single stone occupying the entire sac, and can sometimes be identified as a filling defect on dacryocystography. They can be identified by diagnostic transcanalicular endoscopy, if this is available. At DCR surgery, look for stones in the inferior part of the lacrimal sac and in the upper part of the nasolacrimal duct in middle-aged subjects with a relatively short history of epiphora and acute dacryocystitis. The stones or plaques may be found tucked into a fold or diverticulum in the sac wall.

Figure 5.2
Large lacrimal stone from an inflamed and enlarged sac.

Part B: *Dacryocystorhinostomy*

Dacryocystorhinostomy (DCR) surgery consists of making a permanent opening from the lacrimal sac into the nasal space through which the tears will drain freely, resulting in the relief of epiphora and discharge. Ideally, the common canaliculus will open directly into the nose, with the sac mucosa forming part of the lateral nasal wall.

Indications

Patients with epiphora, mucocoele, or chronic dacryocystitis from stenosis of the nasolacrimal duct with either normal canaliculi or only distal/membranous common canalicular block:

1. Primary acquired nasolacrimal duct obstruction (including functional epiphora from duct narrowing)
2. Secondary acquired nasolacrimal duct obstruction, e.g. post-maxillary or ethmoid sinus surgery, lateral rhinotomy, Wegener's granulomatosis and sarcoidosis
3. Persistent congenital nasolacrimal duct obstruction (see Chapter 4).

Patients with epiphora from canalicular disease require more complex surgery (see Chapter 6):

1. DCR with retrograde canaliculostomy and intubation for mid-canalicular and proximal common canalicular block

2. Canaliculo-DCR for marked proximal common canalicular block
3. Conjunctivo-DCR and Lester–Jones bypass tube if there is less than 8 mm functioning canaliculus.

Lacrimal sac exploration

Examine the lacrimal sac directly at DCR to exclude pathology when there is:

1. Acute/chronic dacryocystitis
2. Suspected lacrimal sac tumour – if a lacrimal sac tumour is found, dacryocystectomy and partial excision of the nasolacrimal duct is indicated
3. Recurrent mucocoele after previous DCR surgery.

Types of DCR

There are two main types of DCR; external and endonasal.

External approach DCR

In this operation, the lacrimal sac and nasal mucosa are approached via a skin incision. A large bony rhinostomy is made between the sac and the nose. An anastomosis is made between the lacrimal sac and nasal mucosa by sutured flaps. The inside of the sac can be explored and adhesions within the sac dissected.

There are two options for the skin incision:

1. Straight side of nose. This is the most common incision, and is a vertical incision made 1 cm away from the medial canthal angle to prevent a bowed scar. The angular vein is safe if a skin flap incision is used.
2. Tear trough. Alternative incision. This is a curved incision in a relaxed skin tension line in the tear trough, over the infero-medial orbital rim, through the skin and orbicularis down to the rim. It starts 2 mm above the medial canthal tendon and avoids the angular vein. It is best done with electrocautery, for example using the Colorado cutting needle. The position of the incision is critical, as too high above the rim could result in division of the nasolacrimal duct during surgery. It is useful for re-do DCR, to avoid the original side of nose incision, or if there has been other medial canthal surgery or radiotherapy. The scar is barely perceptible (see Figure 5.33).

Endonasal (intranasal, transnasal) approach DCR

The nasal mucosa and lacrimal sac are approached via the nose using an endoscope for magnification and illumination. The mucosa is incised and surgically excised or laser ablated. The rhinostomy is usually smaller than that of external DCR. There are no sutured flaps. Tubes are usually used.

There are several different types of endonasal endoscopic DCR:

1. *Endosurgical DCR.* Surgical instruments are used, e.g. Freer's elevator, Blakesley forceps, curette, DCR rongeur and keratome. Alternatively, powered tools are used, e.g. micro-drill or debrider.
2. *Endolaser DCR.* A laser is used to incise and ablate the mucosa and bone. The holmium : YAG or KTP laser are suitable, the latter having greater penetration for bone. The surgery can be entirely by laser.

3. *Endolaser assisted surgical DCR.* Endo-laser DCR often includes the use of endoscopic sinus surgery instruments to remove charred tissue, augment the rhinostomy size and open the lacrimal mucosa.

Silicone intubation in DCR

The indications for temporary silicone intubation are:
1. External DCR when there is:
    *   Canalicular disease, e.g. distal common canalicular membranous occlusion or canalicular DCR
    *   Inflamed sac mucosa, e.g. previous dacryocystitis
    *   Poor flaps, e.g. posterior flaps destroyed and only anterior flaps sutured.
2. Endonasal DCR. There are no sutured flaps.

Rhinostomy size and site

The amount of bone removed and mucosa opened varies between external DCR (large opening) and endoscopic endonasal DCR (smaller opening). The latter is made in the lower sac (Figure 5.3).

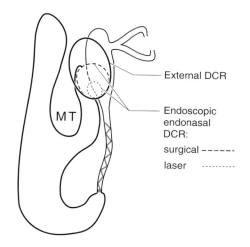

Figure 5.3

Diagram showing the difference in size and location of the per-operative rhinostomy in external DCR compared to endonasal DCR. Note that the endonasal rhinostomy is generally smaller and lower. When healed, there is very little visible difference in size between external and endosurgical DCR, but endolaser DCR may result in a smaller healed ostium.

Healing in DCR

External DCR

The rhinostomy is made through thick maxilla bone and thin lacrimal bone. There is rapid mucosal healing by primary intention where the mucosal edges are sutured, and secondary intention healing where the mucosal edges remain unsutured superiorly and inferiorly. Epithelial continuity is usually complete within 2 weeks of surgery.

Endonasal DCR

The rhinostomy is made mainly through the thin lacrimal bone. The mucosa heals by secondary intention. Epithelial continuity is not complete until about 3–4 weeks after surgery (Figure 5.4).

DCR: historical perspective

Blocked lacrimal systems were treated by probing and syringing in the eighteenth century. Bowman probes were used in the mid-nineteenth century and are still in use today. Serial nasolacrimal duct dilation with probes up to 2 mm in diameter was a standard treatment for epiphora in the first half of the twentieth century. These methods often failed to re-establish nasolacrimal duct patency, and the concept of DCR became established at the end of the nineteenth century and in the early twentieth century. By 1951 external approach DCR was the treatment of choice by ophthalmologists for nasolacrimal duct obstruction, and it has an excellent track record, with surgical success rates greater than 90 per cent. The techniques used now have changed little from those described by Dupuy-Dutemps in 1921, apart from temporary silicone intubation and improved sutures (Figure 5.5).

History of external approach DCR:	
Toti (1904)	Punched out part of lacrimal sac, bone and nasal mucosa
Dupuy-Dutemps and Bourguet (1921)	Addition of sutured mucosal flaps
Hallam (1949)	Intubation with silk suture
Quickert and Dryden (1970)	Intubation with silicone tubes on bodkins

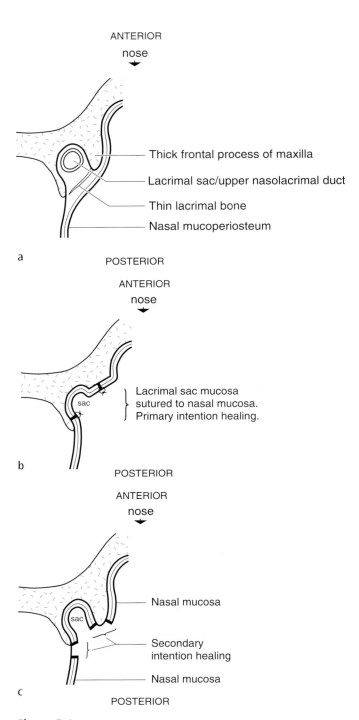

Figure 5.4

a) Diagram showing cross-section at level of lower lacrimal sac/upper nasolacrimal duct. Note the thick maxilla bone antero-medially.

b) The thick maxilla bone as well as thin lacrimal bone is removed in external approach DCR, and the two mucosas are sutured.

c) Mainly thin lacrimal bone is removed in endonasal DCR, and the mucosa are not sutured.

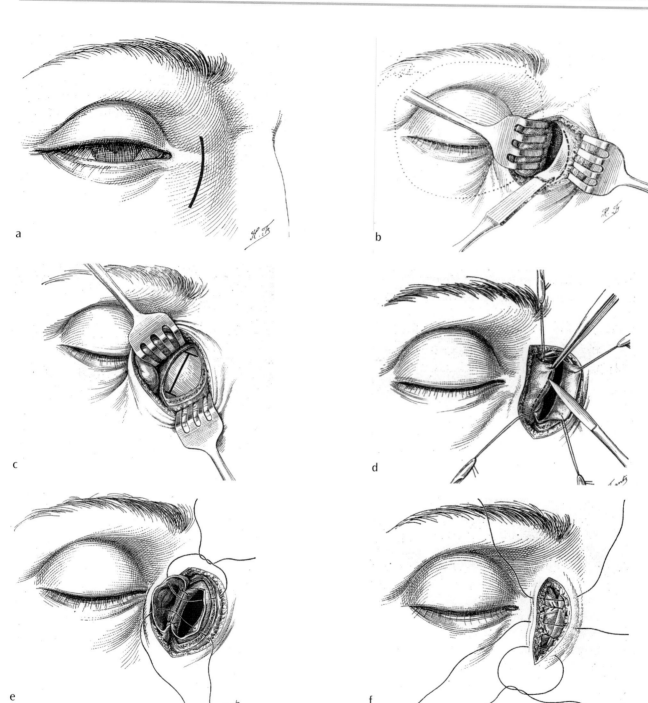

Figure 5.5

Original drawings of external DCR surgery (from Dupuy-Dutemps, 1921).
a) Skin incision.
b) The lacrimal fossa is exposed and the chisel is being used to reduce the anterior lacrimal crest prior to the osteotomy.
c) Following the osteotomy, the exposed nasal mucosa is incised to form the posterior and anterior nasal flaps.
d) The corners of the nasal flaps are on catgut sutures and the lacrimal sac is being incised to create the posterior and anterior lacrimal sac flaps.
e) The posterior mucosal flaps are sutured together and the anterior mucosal flaps are being sutured.
f) The anterior mucosal flaps are sutured together and the skin is being closed with silk sutures.

The endonasal approach (internal, intranasal or transnasal) was described at the end of the nineteenth century by Caldwell (1893), who used an electric drill to resect the medial wall of the nasolacrimal duct from the inferior turbinate up into the lacrimal sac. Other, simpler methods followed in the first half of the twentieth century, often performed by combined otolaryngological/ophthalmological surgeons (Figure 5.6). Illumination and magnification from loups or an operating microscope were poor. Some otolaryngological surgeons continued to perform transnasal dacryocystorhinostomy (Bjork, 1967; Jokinen, 1974; Steadman, 1985), but they were in the minority. The introduction of the rigid endoscope provided the catalyst for endonasal endoscopic dacryocystorhinostomy, often performed jointly by ENT and ophthalmic surgeons. The surgical success rates have tended to be lower than those for external approach DCR.

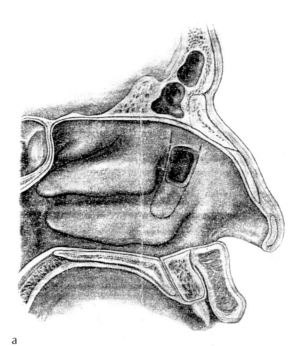

a

History of endonasal non-endoscopic approach DCR:	
Caldwell (1893)	Electric drill medial wall nasolacrimal duct and lacrimal sac
West (1914)	Surgical window resection
Jones (1951)	Intubation with dermal suture
Jones (1962)	Intranasal (non-sutured) mucosal flap and polyethylene tubing

History of endonasal endoscopic DCR:	
McDonogh and Meiring (1989)	Endoscopic endonasal dacryocystorhinostomy
Massaro *et al.* (1990)	Argon laser DCR in cadaver
Metson (1991)	Endoscopic surgical DCR
Woog *et al.* (1993)	Holmium laser assisted DCR

Lacrimal surgery continues to evolve, with many older ideas being re-examined and re-applied using improved instrumentation, especially micro-endoscopes, powered tools and lasers.

Is endonasal DCR any better than external DCR?

They are different operations, with different success rates. It is important to explain to patients the pros and cons of each different type of DCR surgery and their relative surgical success rate. As a guideline, external DCR has a 90–95 per cent success rate, endonasal

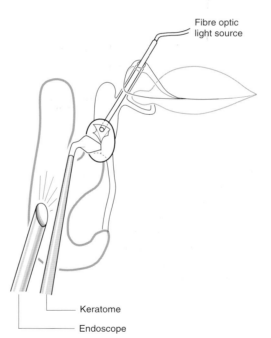

Fibre optic light source

Keratome

Endoscope

b

Figure 5.6

a) Original drawing of early endonasal DCR, showing the window resection over the lower part of the lacrimal sac and upper nasolacrimal duct (from West, 1914, with permission from the Royal Society of Medicine).

b) Diagram showing the current use of an angled keratome to incise the sac mucosa (endoscopic endonasal surgical DCR).

surgical DCR 80–85 per cent, and endonasal laser DCR 70–80 per cent.

Advantages of external DCR:
1. The lacrimal sac is fully exposed, intra-sac pathology identified and the valve of Rosenmuller clearly seen. Membranectomy of the common canalicular opening is possible, as is retrograde intubation.
2. The rhinostomy is large (at least 10 mm), with all the intervening bone and sinus adjacent to the common opening removed; therefore the healed rhinostomy is unlikely to close.
3. Mucosal flaps are sutured and therefore silicone intubation is only used if indicated, as healing is rapid.

Disadvantages of external DCR:
1. Controlled hypotensive general anaesthesia may be contraindicated in elderly frail patients. Local anaesthesia is not always a suitable alternative.
2. Per-operative haemorrhage may impede the view of the common opening and make suturing of the posterior flaps difficult.
3. Surgery is lengthy, up to 60 minutes, depending on the individual surgeon's experience.
4. There is a risk of sump syndrome if the rhinostomy is placed too high in relation to the lacrimal sac. In the sump syndrome, the lacrimal system is patent to syringing but intermittent symptoms of epiphora and stickiness persist because the lacrimal sac cannot drain fully.
5. Re-do surgery may be complicated by excess fibrous tissue within the rhinostomy site and around the sac remnant, which has to be carefully dissected away.
6. The cutaneous scar is occasionally visible.

Advantages of endonasal DCR:
1. Suitable for local anaesthetic day surgery as there is rapid post-operative rehabilitation. Highly suitable for elderly frail patients who would be medically at risk if given a general anaesthesia and a longer operation.
2. There is good haemostasis.
3. Surgery lasts 10–35 minutes.
4. There is no risk of sump syndrome, as the rhinostomy is always adjacent to the lower part of the lacrimal sac.
5. Surgery is localized with very little collateral damage, which makes re-do surgery straightforward, whether by external or endonasal approach.
6. It avoids skin incision and hence risk of a visible facial scar.
7. Patients prefer this operation. Young people wish to avoid the facial scar, and some elderly wish to avoid a general anaesthetic and potentially long operation, despite being informed that the success rates are lower than with external DCR.

Disadvantages of endonasal DCR:
1. There is a learning curve, with new anatomy and instruments, for an ophthalmologist. It is best done in conjunction with an ENT colleague who already has the appropriate expertise and instruments.
2. The cost of endoscopes and instruments is high.
3. Temporary silicone intubation is usually indicated for at least 5 weeks.
4. The inside of the lacrimal sac and common opening is not always visualized.
5. The delicate lacrimal mucosa may be damaged, with resultant scarring.
6. There are lower success rates, due to granuloma and submucosal fibrosis sometimes causing rhinostomy closure.

Assessment of patient for surgery

Non-steroidal anti-inflammatory drugs and anticoagulants will cause excess per-operative bleeding, especially for external DCR. Stop aspirin-containing drugs 2 weeks before surgery, and reduce warfarin so that the INR falls below 2.0 if the medical condition permits. Consult a physician or haematologist if in doubt. There are some conditions, such as a mechanical prosthetic heart valve, in which there may be some risks to the patient in reducing the warfarin to this extent. After discussion with the patient's physician, you may have to admit the patient for intravenous heparin therapy – or opt for endonasal laser DCR.

Many over-the-counter analgesics contain aspirin, e.g. Phensic, and the patient may not be aware of this.

I. External approach DCR

The absolute indication to do an external DCR is a suspected sac neoplasm. Other indications are relative.

Safe guidelines: when to do an external DCR
1. Only one chance.
2. Suspected lacrimal sac tumour (absolute indication).
3. Previous fractured lateral nasal wall with possible bone displacement.
4. Canalicular disease – retrograde canaliculostomy with intubation, canaliculo-DCR or conjunctivo-DCR planned.

5. Sac mucosa – small scarred sac (or inflamed mucosa from previous dacryocystitis), therefore large nasal mucosal flaps required.

6. Nasal mucosa inflamed, with chronic sinusitis, nasal polyps and copious discharge (some surgeons may say this is an indication for endonasal DCR).

Anaesthesia

General

Most surgeons prefer to do external DCR under general anaesthesia. General anaesthetic day case surgery is best done on a morning operating list.

A throat pack or laryngeal mask is required. Good haemostasis is obtained with inhalational agents isofluorane or desfluorane to lower the blood pressure, often with a short-acting beta-blocker (e.g. labetolol) to reduce tachycardia and lower CO_2 levels. The patient is positioned head up (reverse Trendelenberg). Good nasal mucosal vasoconstriction is recommended, using a cocaine 4–10% solution.

Local

This is an alternative for the elderly and frail patient. The drawbacks have been mentioned above. The ocular surface, medial eyelids, medial canthus and anterior lacrimal crest, and nasal mucosa must be anaesthetized. The nasal mucosa must also be decongested (see Figure 5.36).

> **TIPS**
>
> To reduce bleeding:
> 1. *Drugs – avoid aspirin and reduce warfarin if permitted.*
> 2. *Place patient per-operatively with head-up tilt (reverse Trendelenberg).*
> 3. *Control hypotensive general anaesthesia with beta-blockade, or give good infiltration with lidocaine and adrenaline if local anaesthesia.*
> 4. *Vasoconstrict nasal mucosa using cocaine 4–10%.*
> 5. *Per-operatively, use neurosurgical patties soaked in adrenaline 1 in 1000.*
> 6. *Careful surgery – avoid damaging the angular vein by using the skin flap technique or tear trough*

incision. Respect tissue planes and handle tissue gently.

7. *Use traction sutures to reduce orbicularis bleeding.*
8. *Sucker use – use sucker in the non-dominant hand as the second instrument once the lacrimal fossa has been exposed. Place sucker in the posterior nasal space once the nasal mucosa has been opened. If a sucker is still needed as a second instrument, place a second 12 g bronchial sucker in the nose.*
9. *Remove bleeding opened anterior ethmoid mucosa.*
10. *Suture posterior flaps.*

Surgical rules

1. Make the rhinostomy large enough to expose adequate nasal mucosa anteriorly for good flaps – the purpose of the flaps is to enable the common canalicular opening to open freely into the nose.

2. Ensure that no tissue (strands of mucosa, residual ethmoid or maxilla bone) remains medial to the common canalicular opening that could occlude it.

How to avoid post-operative sump syndrome

The sump syndrome can be avoided by aiming the surgery infero-medially from the sac into the nose. This is aided by the correct patient/surgeon positioning during surgery. The surgeon sits diagonally, not absolutely at the side of the patient or at the head. The theatre nurse sits on the other side of the patient, and the assistant at the head of the table. For training purposes, the resident should look down into the wound from over the surgeon's shoulder in order to see the same view.

> **TIP**
>
> *The surgeon should sit and aim infero-medially to avoid sump syndrome.*

Standard external DCR – surgical steps

> **Surgical steps:**
> 1. Skin incision
> 2. Expose ascending process of maxilla and lacrimal fossa
> 3. Rhinostomy ± anterior ethmoidectomy
> 4. Create mucosal flaps and intubate
> 5. Skin closure.

Skin incision

> **Instruments for skin incision:**
> - Marker pen and calliper
> - No. 15 blade on Barde Parker handle or Colorado needle
> - St Martin's toothed forceps
> - Westcott's curved scissors
> - Straight, blunt scissors
> - Moorfield's non-toothed forceps
> - Silk traction sutures (cutting needle), e.g. Ethicon 4/0 Mersilk W606 or W501
> - Castroviejo needle holder
> - Five artery clips
> - Rollet's rugine.
>
> NB: Lay the instruments out in the order they will be used.

Procedure: Use either the straight lateral side of nose or tear trough incision. The straight side of nose incision is made vertically, anteriorly (medially) to the angular vein, initially through the skin only and *not* straight down through the orbicularis to the bone. Instead a skin flap is raised and a skin pocket created, which avoids the vein. This incision is recommended (Figure 5.7). For the tear trough incision, see Figure 5.33.

Steps:

- Mark the vertical skin incision with a pen. Use a calliper to measure distances if necessary. The incision is placed 10 mm from the medial canthal angle and extends approximately 2 mm above and 10 mm below the horizontal inter-canthal line. Its length is 12–15 mm in adults and 6–8 mm in children. Use the blade or Colorado needle to incise the skin only (Figure 5.8).
- Raise the skin flap by dissecting between the skin and vein/orbicularis, in a natural tissue plane. Use curved scissors to separate the orbicularis/skin attachments. Use straight, blunt scissors to divide

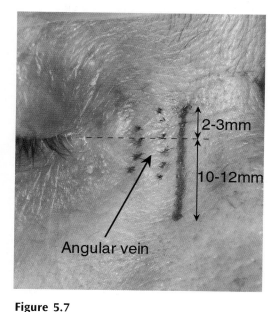

Figure 5.7

External DCR lateral side of nose skin incision. The angular vein lies medial to the incision.

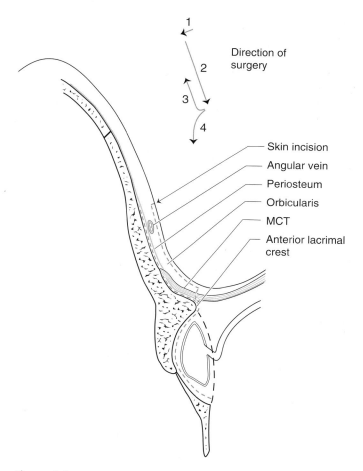

Figure 5.8

Diagram showing the external DCR stepped skin incision. After the skin incision, the skin flap is raised. The maxilla is cleaned, then the lacrimal fossa is entered. MCT = medial canthal tendon.

the pretarsal and preseptal orbicularis fibres at the anterior lacrimal crest. Reflect the lateral skin flap laterally on two traction sutures secured firmly to the drapes (Figure 5.9).

● Identify the superficial medial canthal tendon (MCT) and divide all or lower two-thirds with a blade or Rollet's rugine. Place the lateral cut end on a small marker suture.

● Use the Rollet's rugine to divide the periosteum along the anterior lacrimal crest. Lift the periosteum anterior off the ascending process of the maxilla – aim for the bridge of the nose. This should be at least 10 mm anteriorly in order to create a good-sized rhinostomy, and hence good-sized nasal mucosal flaps (Figure 5.9).

● Place three 4.0 black silk traction sutures around the medial orbicularis/vein/skin and secure them tightly to the drapes. The lowest traction suture is called the 'white nose' or 'break nose' suture, as it is secured very tightly over the nose, leaving a temporary indent. Bend the needle with an artery clip in order to take a short deep bite of orbicularis (Figure 5.10).

● The suture of Notha (emissary vein) is anterior to the anterior lacrimal crest and may bleed – use the sucker or apply bone wax.

See Figure 5.11.

Ascending process of maxilla and lacrimal fossa exposure

Specific anatomy: See Figure 5.12.

> **Instruments to enter lacrimal fossa (Figure 5.13):**
> - Sucker
> - Rollet's rugine (optional: Hill's periosteal elevator)
> - Traquair's periosteal elevator.

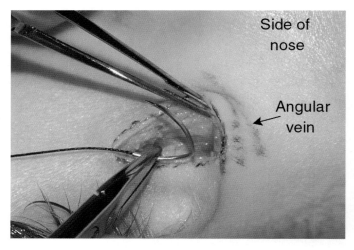

Figure 5.10

A bent needle fits easily into the wound. (Left tear trough incision from above, hence angular vein medial to incision).

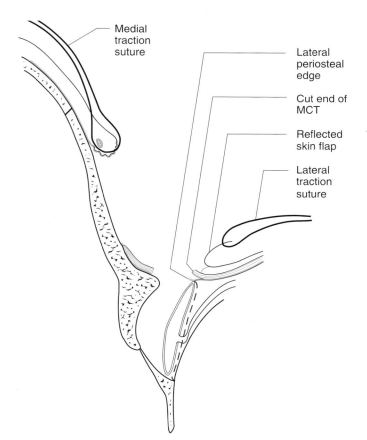

Figure 5.9

Diagram showing traction sutures and exposed lacrimal fossa.

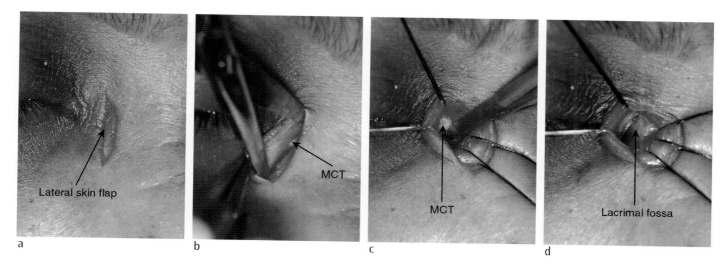

Figure 5.11

a)   Skin incision on lateral side of nose.
b)   Skin flap created anterior to orbicularis, angular vein and MCT.
c)   Good view of MCT in pocket created.
d)   Lacrimal fossa exposed.

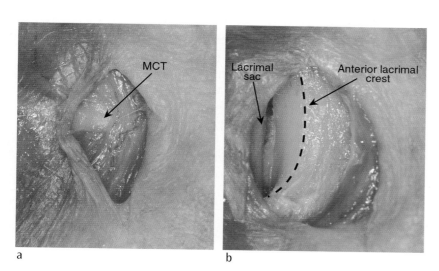

Figure 5.12

Right lacrimal anatomy.

a)   The superficial part of the medial canthal tendon (MCT) lies immediately beneath the skin, inserting into the ascending process of the maxilla. Note its free lower edge.

b)   The anterior lacrimal crest on the maxilla bone lies beneath the orbicularis muscle. It is a clearly defined bony ridge, more prominent inferiorly. The periosteum has to be opened to expose the lacrimal fossa. The suture of Notha lies anterior to the anterior lacrimal crest.

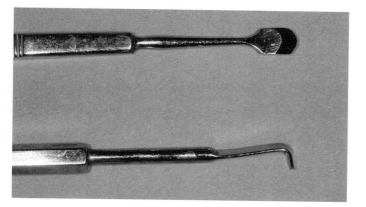

Figure 5.13

Top, Rollet's rugine; bottom, Traquair's periosteal elevator.

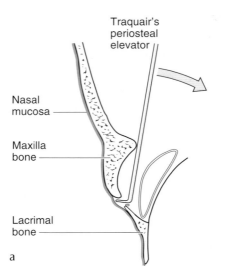
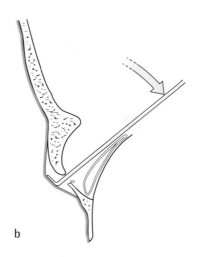

a

b

Figure 5.14

a)   Traquair's periosteal elevator is held vertically as its tip penetrates the thin lacrimal bone.

b)   Once through the bone, the handle is swung laterally so that the tip does not damage the nasal mucosa and can effectively elevate the nasal mucosa off the bone.

Procedure: Expose as much bone anterior to the anterior lacrimal crest as possible. Use the traction sutures and a squint hook to reflect the orbicularis anterior off the bone. Use the sucker in the non-dominant hand throughout to aspirate blood and reflect tissue.

Steps:

● Reflect the periosteum and orbicularis laterally and identify the lacrimal sac. It is sometimes useful to put a marker suture on the edge of the reflected periosteum for later orientation.

● Enter the lacrimal fossa with Rollet's rugine – there is a natural plane between the sac and the bony fossa. Be careful not to penetrate the thin lacrimal

bone in the lacrimal fossa yet, or damage the lacrimal sac. Use the sucker to reflect the sac and upper part of the nasolacrimal duct gently and laterally.

● Identify the vertical bone suture in the lacrimal fossa using the Traquair's periosteal elevator and penetrate the thin lacrimal bone superiorly, posterior to the suture. Always use the short end of the periosteal elevator if they are different sizes. Initially hold the Traquair handle vertically so that the tip enters at right angles through the bone, and once it is in swing the handle laterally 90° so that the tip is behind and parallel to the bone and cannot damage the nasal mucosa (Figures 5.14, 5.15).

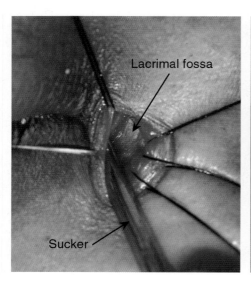

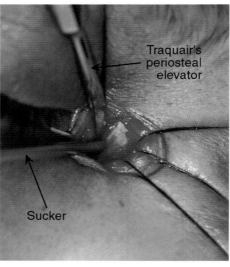

Figure 5.15

a)   The sucker is in the lacrimal fossa.

b)   With sucker in one hand, the Traquair's periosteal elevator probes through the bony suture and outfractures a small amount of thin lacrimal bone.

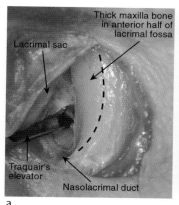
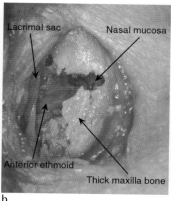
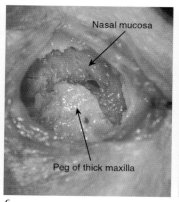
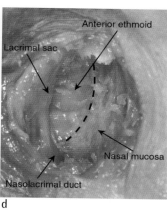

a   b   c   d

Figure 5.16

Right lacrimal anatomy.

a) The thick maxilla bone forms the anterior half of the lacrimal fossa, with the thin lacrimal bone posteriorly, separated by a vertical suture. The anterior lacrimal crest extends inferiorly and laterally, anterior to the commencement of the nasolacrimal duct, and is continuous with the medial part of the inferior orbital rim. The ascending process of the maxilla bone is particularly thick inferiorly.

b) Anterior ethmoid air cells lie between the lacrimal sac and the nose in the superior posterior lacrimal fossa in over 90 per cent of cadavers.

c) The undersurface of the nasal mucosa is visible when the ascending process of the maxilla bone is removed. Note the thickness of the lower part of the anterior lacrimal crest, seen here as a thick bony peg.

d) The relations of the lacrimal sac, anterior ethmoid and nasal mucosa become evident when the thick peg of ascending process of the maxilla is removed. The anterior ethmoid air cells have thin mucosa and bony septa, which run antero-posteriorly. In this dissection, the lacrimal sac and duct is lateral, anterior ethmoid central and undersurface of nasal mucosa medial.

Rhinostomy

Specific anatomy: See Figure 5.16.

> **Instruments for rhinostomy (Figure 5.17):**
> * Traquair's periosteal elevator
> * Kerrison bone punches – up-cut in small, medium and large sizes
> * Bone nibblers, e.g. Beyer punch
> * Optional: hammer, chisel and bone wax.

Procedure: Make an initial C-shaped rhinostomy which enables easy removal of the thickest part of the maxilla inferiorly. Ethmoid air cells between the lacrimal fossa and nasal mucosa are removed. The rhinostomy should be large enough to accommodate a large finger or thumb (Figure 5.18).

Steps:

* Use the Traquair's periosteal elevator to separate the nasal mucosa and bone by running it superior and inferior in the bony suture, and gently pushing the

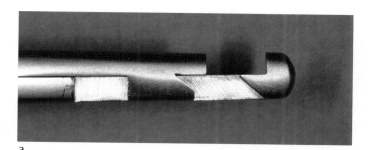

a

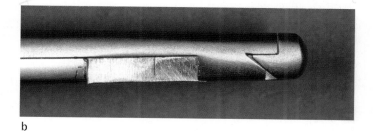

b

Figure 5.17

a) Up-cut Kerrison bone punch with 90° bite – tip open.
b) Tip of punch closed.

i)   ii)   iii)   iv)   v)

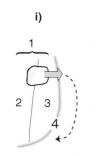
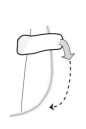
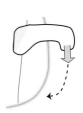
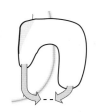
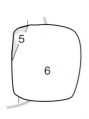

Figure 5.18

Diagrams showing direction of rongeur during rhinostomy. Start high in the lacrimal fossa, work anterior then inferior (C-shape), and then lastly remove the thick inferior peg.

KEY

1 Lacrimal fossa
2 Lacrimal bone
3 Maxilla bone
4 Anterior lacrimal crest

5 Anterior ethmoid
6 Undersurface of
  nasal mucosa

mucosa away. Never have anything in the nose (nasal pack or instrument) that could push the mucosa towards the bone whilst doing the rhinostomy.

- Enlarge the initial lacrimal bone fracture to make an adequately large space to insert the bone punch. Pull the Traquairs' towards you to outfracture little fragments of lacrimal bone. Use the sucker in the non-dominant hand to reflect the sac laterally and aspirate blood.

- Use the rongeurs to make the C-shaped rhinostomy anteriorly into the maxilla, starting superiorly. Initially go anteriorly towards the bridge of the nose,

then inferiorly, and finally posteriorly. The thickest bone is inferior – if this is weakened it becomes easy to remove with a rongeur or bone clipper (Figure 5.20). The rhinostomy should extend from the fundus of the sac superiorly and the posterior lacrimal crest posteriorly. It should go at least 10 mm anteriorly towards the bridge of the nose, and inferiorly including the upper part of the medial nasolacrimal canal and the hamular process. The round-shaped rhinostomy should measure 10–18 mm in diameter. The assistant retracts the medial orbicularis with a squint hook to help expose the maxilla for removal.

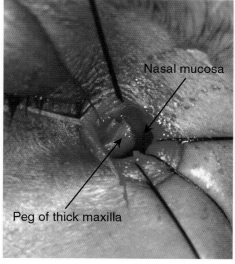

Nasal mucosa

Peg of thick maxilla

a

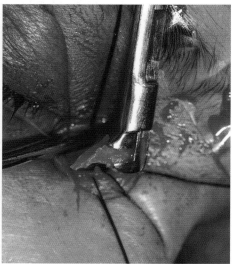

b

Figure 5.19 (right side)

a) C-shaped rhinostomy has been made and the thick peg of maxilla remains inferior.

b) The peg is removed using the rongeurs. Note that the peg includes part of the anterior lacrimal fossa close to the lower end of the lacrimal sac/upper nasolacrimal duct.

TIP

Keep elevating the nasal mucosa off the bone by alternate use of rongeur and periosteal elevator in order to keep the nasal mucosa intact. The assistant or theatre nurse cleans the rongeur of entrapped bone after each bite, using a damp gauze square, and holds the Traquair's periosteal elevator for exchange.

- Excise anterior ethmoid mucosa (this bleeds) and thin ethmoid bone fragments. Ensure that the nasal mucosa is also free of all small fragments of bone, using Moorfield's forceps to feel for small bone fragments and remove them. The rhinostomy will expose the undersurface of the nasal mucosa, seen as a grey mucosal sheet.

TIP

Differentiate between ethmoid and nasal mucosa. Nasal mucosa is grey and thick. Anterior ethmoid mucosa is pink/white, thin, and more prone to bleeding.

TIP

Do not confuse entering the ethmoid for entering the nose. If in doubt, place a Stallard instrument in the nasal space, directed up towards the rhinostomy – it should be seen indenting the nasal mucosa. Alternatively, use a cotton bud. Do not use the sucker. Placing an instrument in the nasal space will also show whether nasal mucosa has been inadvertently lost during the rhinostomy.

Create mucosal flaps and intubate

Specific anatomy: See Figure 5.20.

Instruments to create flaps and intubate:
• Nettleship punctal dilator
• Bowman probes size 0/00 and 1/2
• No. 11 blade, or paracentesis knife
• Werb right-angled sac scissors or Westcott scissors
• Stallard's blunt lacrimal dissector
• O'Donoghue silicone tubes on metal bodkins
• St Martin's toothed forceps
• Curved artery clip
• 6.0 absorbable suture on half circle spatula needle, e.g. Ethicon 6/0 Vicryl W9566 or Davis and Geck 4567-13 Dexon 'S'
• Barraquer needle holder
• Optional for securing tubes: Ligaclips and applicator or Watzke sleeve.

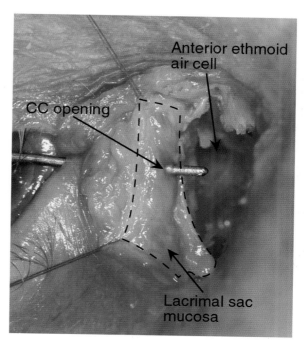

Figure 5.20

The common canalicular opening lies between the upper third and lower two-thirds of the lacrimal sac. The sac/nasolacrimal duct junction lies just within the upper part of the nasolacrimal canal. The normal lacrimal sac mucosa is smooth and pale pink. There is a single common canalicular (CC) opening in over 80 per cent of adult lacrimal sacs. The anterior ethmoid lies between the lacrimal sac and nose in over 90 per cent of cadavers.

Procedure: Make the lacrimal flaps first. If tubes are inserted, they will help retract the lacrimal mucosa safely. Make the nasal mucosal flaps second, because once cut they bleed. Aim to suture both the posterior and anterior flaps. Sometimes it is not possible to suture the posterior flaps because of bleeding or mucosal loss, in which case a large anterior flap is effective (Figure 5.22).

Steps:

- Dilate the lower punctum with the Nettleship dilator and then insert the Bowman probe size 1 along the inferior canaliculus into the sac, tenting up its medial wall.
- Incise the medial sac wall vertically using a paracentesis knife or no. 11 blade. Extend the superior and inferior ends of the incision anteriorly and posteriorly to create the flaps. Ensure that the full thickness of the lacrimal wall has been incised,

and not just the overlying thin adventitia, by directly inspecting the Bowman probe inside the sac. Place 6.0 absorbable sutures on the two corners of the anterior flap and reflect it laterally.

● Look inside the sac for folds, diverticulae, dacryoliths, polyps and other pathology. If there is a membrane or fibrous mucosal fold over the common opening that held up passage of the probe, do a membrectomy with Vannas' scissors. Use the microscope or an endoscope for a better view.

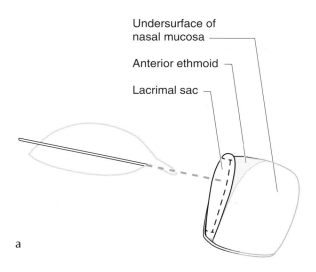

a

Lacrimal flaps

Relative sizes of anterior and posterior lacrimal flaps:
1. If the lacrimal sac is of a normal size, the anterior flaps are made the same size as the posterior flaps, 1 : 1, anterior : posterior.
2. If the lacrimal sac is very small, aim for a good sized anterior flap, 2 : 1, anterior : posterior.
3. If there is little remaining nasal mucosa (e.g. it has been lost during rhinostomy), first try and find some anteriorly by enlarging the rhinostomy. If there is still inadequate nasal mucosa, the lacrimal sac mucosa will form the entire anterior flap (sutured to the undersurface of the medial periosteum/orbicularis), therefore 3 : 1 or 4 : 1, anterior : posterior. The posterior flap is omitted.
4. If there is a large lacrimal sac (e.g. a mucocoele or diverticulum is present), it is sometimes necessary to excise part of the lacrimal mucosa so that the sutured flap does not flop back inwards and obstruct the common opening. The anterior flap will still be larger than the posterior because sac enlargement occurs anteriorly.
5. If the lacrimal mucosa is badly damaged during incision, excise loose fragments and aim for a large flap derived from anterior or posterior nasal mucosa.

If intubation is planned, insert the O'Donoghue silicone tubes now and use the tubes clipped back laterally onto the drapes, to reflect the sac mucosa open and provide greater access to the nasal mucosa (Figure 5.22).

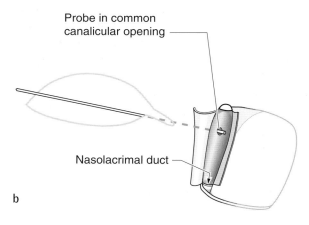

b

Figure 5.21

Diagrams showing how to make lacrimal flaps.
a) Bowman probe tenting up lacrimal sac mucosa for cut down.
b) Lacrimal sac flaps cut and common canaliculus internal opening visible.

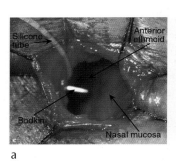

a

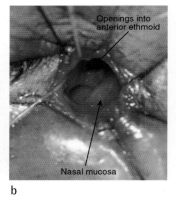

b

Figure 5.22

a) The bodkin is directed infero-medially and seen emerging from the internal opening. The first part of the silicone tube is pulled through and reflected laterally to keep the sac retracted. The second bodkin is pulled through.
b) The ethmoid is opened and the nasal mucosa is visible.

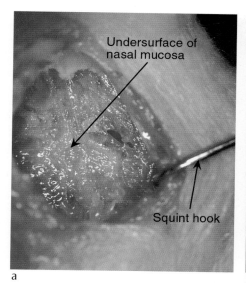
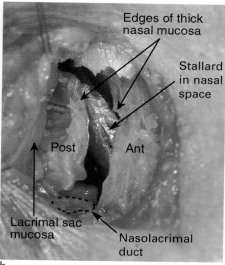
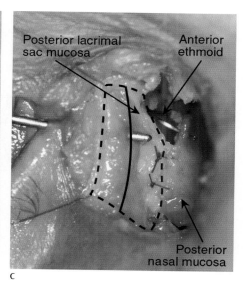

a   b   c

Figure 5.23

a) Beneath the ascending process of the maxilla lies the undersurface of the nasal mucosa. It is thick and grey. A squint hook reflects the orbicularis and skin anterior.

b) The nasal mucosa has been opened to demonstrate the nasal space. The Stallard seeker placed in the nose confirms that the mucosa demonstrated is nasal mucosa and *not* anterior ethmoid (e.g. a large agger nasi).

c) Lacrimal sac and nasal mucosa are separated by the anterior ethmoid. The greater the amount of ethmoid between the sac and nose, the greater the distance between the common opening and the sagittal plane of the lateral nasal wall. Here, the posterior nasal mucosa has been lined up with the posterior sac mucosa showing intervening ethmoid.

Retrograde intubation may be required if there is proximal or mid-canalicular obstruction.

Nasal flaps

Specific anatomy: See Figure 5.23.

Procedure: Aim to make both anterior and posterior nasal flaps. The greater the area of nasal mucosa exposed, the more likely it is that you will be able to fashion two flaps.

> **Relative sizes of anterior and posterior nasal flaps:**
> 1. The anterior flap is the same or larger than the posterior, 1 : 1 or 2 : 1, anterior : posterior.
> 2. If there is only a very small amount of nasal mucosa, either as a result of trauma or a very low agger nasi, create a single anterior nasal flap.
> 3. If the nasal mucosa has been damaged anteriorly, only a posterior flap will be possible. The anterior flap will therefore be made from the lacrimal sac mucosa only.

Insert Stallard's instrument into the nose medially to the exposed nasal mucosa and repeat the incision. Cut down onto the Stallard with a paracentesis knife or no. 11 or 15 blade. If using a long blade, avoid inadvertently cutting the skin with the upper part of the blade. Use Werb's angled or Westcott's curved scissors for the horizontal cuts. If a single anterior flap of nasal mucosa is planned, incise the nasal mucosa more posteriorly (Figures 5.24, 5.25).

Suture the posterior flaps

At this point the posterior flaps are usually sutured together with interrupted or continuous 6.0 absorbable suture.

TIP

Keep both ends of the suture out of the wound at all times and keep the Barraquer needle holder and St Martin's forceps clean of dried blood by wiping them frequently with a damp gauze square.

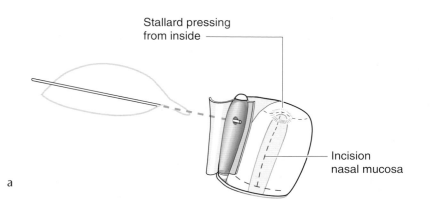

Stallard pressing
from inside

Incision
nasal mucosa

a

Figure 5.24

Diagrams showing how to make nasal flaps.
a) Stallard instrument indenting nasal
    mucosa, for cut down.
b) Nasal mucosal anterior and posterior
    flaps have been prepared. The posterior
    nasal flap is sutured to the posterior
    lacrimal flap.

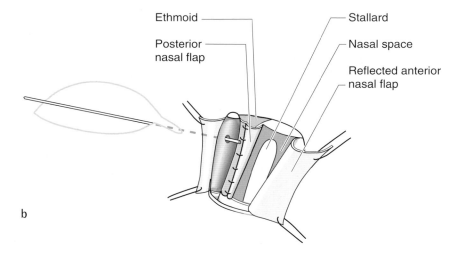

Ethmoid

Stallard

Posterior
nasal flap

Nasal space

Reflected anterior
nasal flap

b

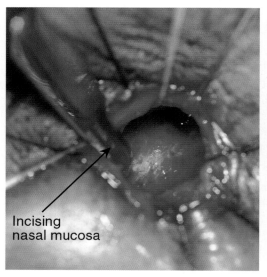

Incising
nasal mucosa

a

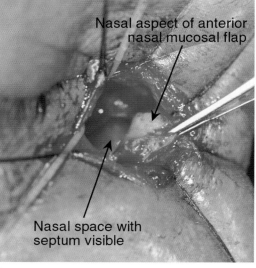

Nasal aspect of anterior
nasal mucosal flap

Nasal space with
septum visible

b

Figure 5.25

a) The nasal mucosa is
    incised.
b) View of the nasal
    space and reflected
    anterior nasal mucosal
    flap.

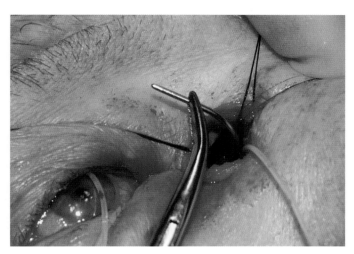

Figure 5.26

The bodkin is pulled out of the DCR wound.

Silicone intubation

Procedure: The tubes are often inserted before creating the nasal flaps, as shown in Figures 5.26, 5.27 and 5.28.

Steps:

- Dilate the punctum with the Nettleship dilator.
- Bend the metal bodkin and insert it gently through the canaliculus. Grasp it within the wound with a curved artery clip and bring it out.
- Repeat with the second bodkin.
- Cut off both bodkins and leave the ends long.
- Tie the silicone tubes together with several knots, Ligaclips or a Watzke sleeve, or a combination of these. Ensure that the tie is not going to lie close to the rhinostomy site (and risk later impaction) by tying the tubes outside the wound and level with the bridge of the nose, over an instrument.

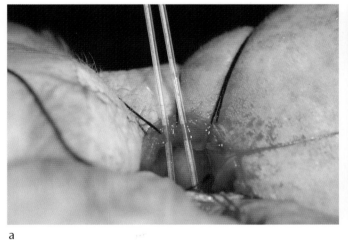

a

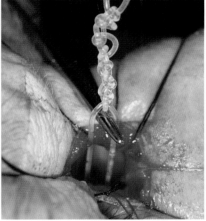

b

Figure 5.27

Secure the tubes.
a) Both ends are held vertically above the wound.
b) They are tied together over an instrument so that no knots or ties will lie within the rhinostomy once inside the nose.

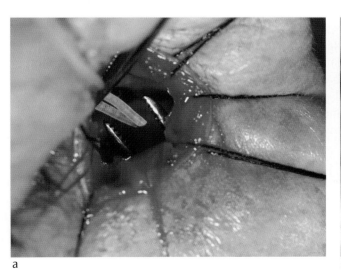

a

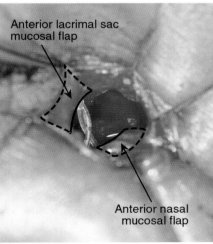

Anterior lacrimal sac mucosal flap

Anterior nasal mucosal flap

b

Figure 5.28

a) The tube ends are directed into the wound and caught by an artery clip placed within the nose.
b) Part of the posterior sutured flap is seen with the tubes across the DCR opening. The tubes pass from the internal opening and into the nose. Next the anterior flaps can be sutured.

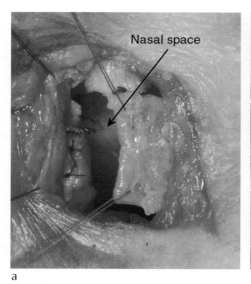

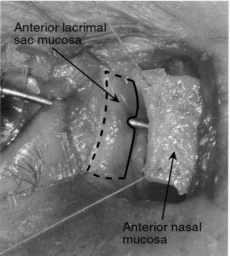

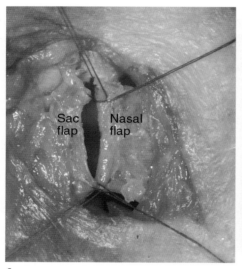

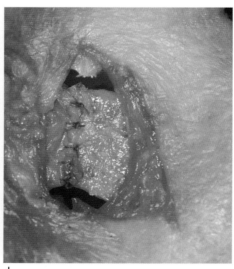

Figure 5.29

a) The nasal mucosa lining the ascending frontal process of the maxilla is thick and strong. In comparison, the lacrimal sac mucosa is thinner.

b) The common canalicular opening is 3–5 mm below the apex and divides the sac into anterior and posterior parts.

c) The mucosa are stretched across the space between the sac and the nasal space usually occupied by bone.

d) Maxilla bone edges are visible above and below.

● Pass the tubes down into the nose by holding the two ends together with forceps within the wound. Place a curved artery clip up through the nostril into the deep part of the wound to catch the ends and pull them down back through the nose and out of the nostril.

Suture the anterior flaps
Specific anatomy: See Figure 5.29.

Procedure: Suture together the anterior flaps as for the posterior, using either interrupted or continuous 6.0 absorbable suture. If interrupted sutures, start by pre-placing the suture at each corner of the anterior nasal flap and one on the anterior lacrimal flap. Understand that the lacrimal sac and nasal mucosal flaps are not always exactly adjacent horizontally, but are often at different heights, with the nasal mucosal flap being lower (Figure 5.30).

Skin closure

Procedure: For the skin sutures use 6.0 monofilament, e.g. Prolene or Novafil (Davis and Geck 4567-13), in adults; use 7.0 absorbable suture in children.

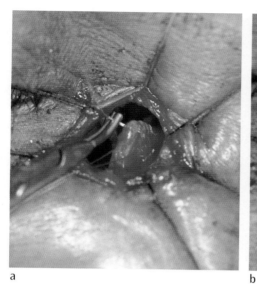

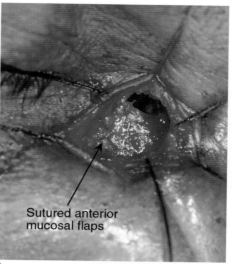

a

b

Sutured anterior
mucosal flaps

Figure 5.30

a) The anterior flap is sutured anterior to the tubes. The sac was small, but plenty of nasal mucosa was available. There is an inferior pre-placed suture on the nasal flap, and the superior one is being placed.

b) The anterior lacrimal and nasal mucosal flaps are anastomosed with five interrupted sutures. Alternative is a continuous suture in each flap. The sutured edges will heal rapidly by primary intention. The free upper mucosal edge visible will heal by secondary intention.

Avoid orbicularis sutures. Repair the MCT with one 6.0 absorbable suture, or leave it if there is no displacement. The muscle layer is self-sealing if the skin flap incision was used; simply reposition the orbicularis over the anterior mucosal flaps. Close the skin (Figure 5.31).

Cut the tubes to the correct length in the vestibule of the nose, whilst on slight stretch, making sure that the tube is not too tight at the medial canthus. Optional: pack the nose with a dry sponge nasal pack coated with chloramphenicol ointment.

Alternative tear trough skin incision (Figure 5.32)

Exploration of inferior medial canthal masses: Although most of these will be large lacrimal sac mucocoeles, not all masses in this area arise from the lacrimal sac. The mass may be extrinsic to the sac. A tear trough incision is suitable (Figures 5.33, 5.34).

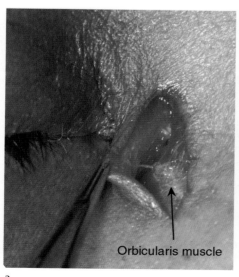

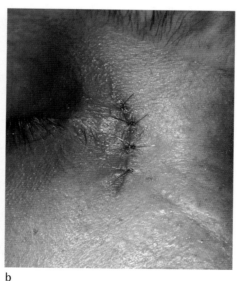

a

b

Orbicularis muscle

Figure 5.31

a) The orbicularis has been repositioned over the anterior sutured flaps. The MCT is not displaced. The skin flap is then repositioned medially.

b) The wound is closed with interrupted sutures. A continuous suture is equally good.

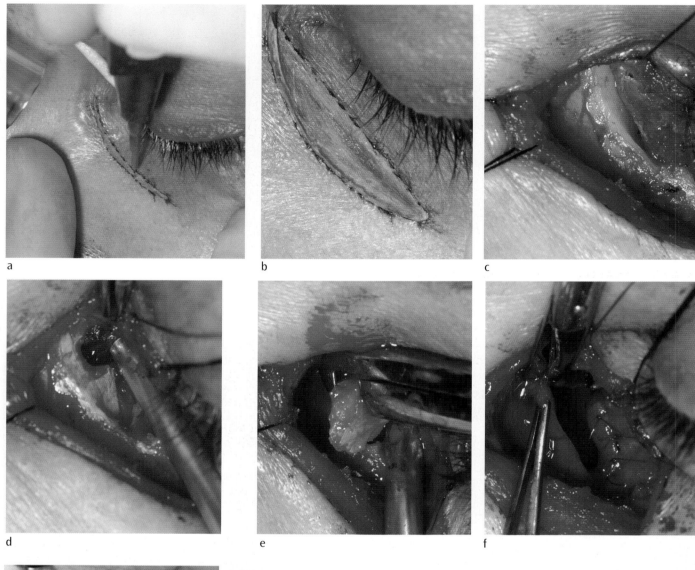

Figure 5.32

Tear trough incision, external approach DCR.

a)   Curved skin incision made with Colorado needle from MCT (posterior to angular vein) to infero-medial orbital rim (skin on stretch).

b)   Skin–orbicularis incision.

c)   Lower part of anterior lacrimal crest and medial inferior orbital rim exposed. **NB**: The sac–nasolacrimal duct junction is adjacent, and it is essential to keep the dissection onto the bony rim to avoid inadvertent laceration of the duct.

d)   There is easy access to the lacrimal fossa, and a C-shaped rhinostomy is made as before. Rhinostomy is just started here.

e)   Once adequate bone has been removed with the rongeurs, there is a good view onto the undersurface of the nasal mucosa.

f)   The posterior flaps are sutured with four or five interrupted 6.0 absorbable sutures.

g)   After tubes have been passed, the anterior flaps are sutured in the normal fashion. The skin incision is then closed with interrupted or continuous 6.0 monofilament as before.

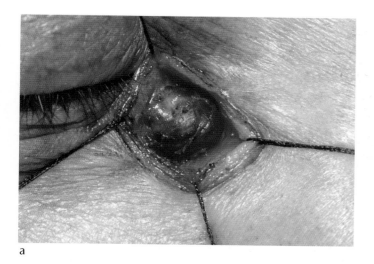 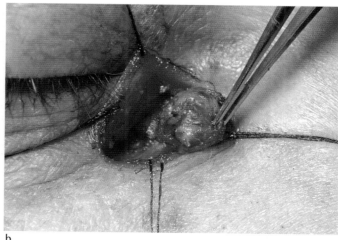

Figure 5.33 Tear trough incision, exploration of mass.

a) Haemangioma exposed, extrinsic to the sac.
b) After diathermy to its stalk, it shrinks and is easily removed.

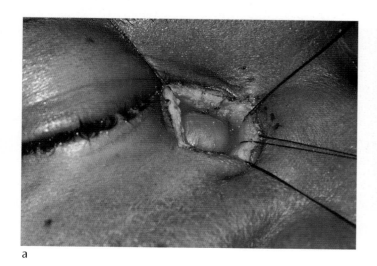 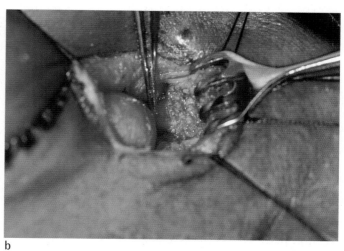

Figure 5.34 Tear trough incision.

a) In this re-do DCR, there is a non-reducible mucocoele.
b) The mucocoele originates from the lacrimal sac. It is completely partitioned off from the sac remnant and is separate from the scar tissue filling the original rhinostomy.

II. Endonasal endoscopic DCR

Endonasal DCR is done under general or local anaesthesia.

Anaesthesia

General

Even under general anaesthesia, the nasal mucosa must be decongested. The options include:

1. Co-phenylcaine Forte nasal spray before nasal packing
2. Guttae phenylephrine 2.5 or 10% on cotton buds, or cocaine 4 or 10% solution nasal on neurosurgical patties or sponge (some surgeons avoid cocaine ointment as this may cloud the endoscope)
3. Moffat's solution, which contains cocaine and adrenaline and is administered directly into the nasal space with the head tipped right back, by the anaesthetist, after the patient is induced.
4. During surgery, adrenaline 1:1000 is applied to the nasal mucosa at the start of the procedure and as necessary.

Local

In addition to nasal mucosal decongestion, the following tissues are anaesthetized prior to surgery:

1. Ocular surface – topical guttae amethocaine.
2. Medial upper and lower eyelids, anterior lacrimal crest and lacrimal fossa – lidocaine 2% and adrenaline 1:200 000. Use either a medial peribulbar or a single horizontal medial canthal angle injection for the anterior lacrimal crest and fossa; the latter avoids the risk of temporary diplopia (Figure 5.36).
3. Nasal mucosa
   - Pre-operative: Apply co-phenylcaine Forte nasal spray to septum, middle turbinate and nasal vestibule. Dose: Up to five squirts for adults, three squirts for 8–12-year-olds, two squirts for 4–8-year-olds, and one squirt for 2–4-year-olds. Alternatively, 1 ml cocaine 4–10% may be applied on a nasal sponge or neurosurgical patties to the nasal space, not forgetting the nasal vestibule via which the intruments pass. NB: Nasal local anaesthesia reaches the back of the throat; therefore warn the patient not to eat or drink anything for 1 hour after application. Reduce the amount of anaesthetic reaching the throat by sitting the patient up with the neck flexed (i.e. chin on chest) or lying the patient flat with the head tilted back.
   - Per-operative: Apply 1 ml adrenaline 1:1000 applied as required to the middle turbinate and meatus. Inject the lateral nasal wall and middle turbinate with bupivicaine 2% and adrenaline 1:80 000 in a 2 ml syringe, using a 20 g spinal needle, if required.

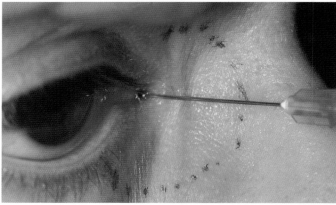

a

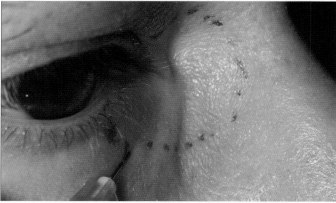

b

Figure 5.35

Local anaesthesia.
a) Right DCR. Area of eyelids, lacrimal fossa and ascending process of maxilla to be anaesthetized is demarcated. Vertical superficial peribulbar block medial to the caruncle, 1.5 ml is injected (can cause temporary diplopia). A single horizontal medial canthal angle injection is better.
b) Inject medial canthus and anterior lacrimal crest (1.5 ml) and upper and lower eyelids (0.5 ml each).

Co-phenylcaine Forte spray contains:
- Lignocaine hydrochloride 5%
- Phenylephrine hydrochloride 0.5%
- Benzalkonium chloride 0.1%

Moffats' solution contains:
- 1 ml adrenaline 1:1000
- 1 ml cocaine solution hcl 10%
- 2 ml sodium bicarbonate
- 16 ml saline 0.9%.

Getting started with endonasal DCR

Endonasal surgery is most commonly performed by an otolaryngologist and an ophthalmologist together. The ophthalmologist initially looks after the upper part of the lacrimal drainage system, but can be trained to do the endonasal part.

TIPS

re endonasal surgeon–patient positioning:
- *Operate from the right side, whether doing a right or left endonasal DCR.*
- *Hold the endoscope in the left hand and instruments in the right hand (reverse only if strongly left handed). Use the left eye to look through the endoscope if possible, unless the right eye is strongly dominant.*
- *Tilt the patient's head towards the surgeon, so that the endoscope easily lies close to the middle meatus.*
- *Either work through the endoscope (head down, direct view) or from the TV screen (head up, indirect view). It is possible for the surgeon to work under direct view while the theatre staff watch on the TV screen, using a split beam adaptor or special camera.*
- *Keep the tip of the endoscope clean by wiping off mucus or blood with a dry gauze and dipping it in an anti-fog solution.*

TIPS

for the surgeon inserting the light pipe:
- *The best position to insert the light pipe is to stand at the top of the patient's head. Once the light pipe is in the lacrimal sac it must be held still unless the endonasal surgeon asks that it be wiggled around. The light pipe holder should be able to see the TV screen fairly easily to check the position.*
- *Avoid orbital fat prolapse into the nose by never letting go of the light pipe – if it partially falls out and is pushed back in without the eyelid being properly stretched the canaliculus may be kinked posterior to the sac, resulting in a falsely positioned beacon posterior to the lacrimal sac, with the risk of canalicular damage and fat prolapse.*

TIPS

for the endonasal surgeon:
- *Respect the nasal mucosa and avoid inadvertent mucosal damage, which could lead to swelling and later synaechiae.*
- *Try and keep the endoscope in the nose all the time, only removing it to defog or clean.*
- *Be careful not to damage the vestibule when inserting and removing instruments.*
- *Hold all second instruments below the endoscope.*

i) Endonasal surgical DCR

The standard instruments depend on which type of endonasal surgical DCR is being done – simple surgical, extended surgical or power tool assisted.

Instruments for endosurgical DCR (Figure 5.36):
- Nettleship dilator
- Vitrectomy light pipe
- 0, 30 or 45° Hopkins endoscope with light source, camera and screen
- Freer's elevator
- Blakesley forceps, straight and up-biting
- Thru-cut Blakesley forceps, straight and up-biting
- Kuhn spoons
- J-curette
- Traquair's periosteal elevator
- Kerrison rongeur, up-biting
- Power drill
- Turbinate scissors
- Keratome
- Short O'Donoghue tubes (bodkins 30 mm long)
- Artery clip.

Steps:
1. Insert light pipe and inject nasal mucosa with local anaesthesia
2. Incise/excise nasal mucosa
3. Remove bone
4. Incise lacrimal sac mucosa
5. Pass and secure O'Donoghue silicone tubes.

Insert light pipe

- Dilate either the upper or lower punctum and insert the light pipe, first vertically and then horizontally, along the canaliculus into the sac. Whilst inserting the pipe horizontally, hold the eyelid on lateral stretch to keep the canaliculus straight.
- Once in the sac (firm stop of medial bony wall), swing the pipe round to an angle between 45 to 70° from the horizontal line, held flat against the frontal

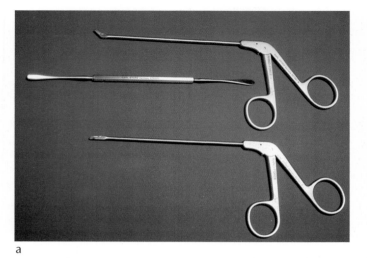

a

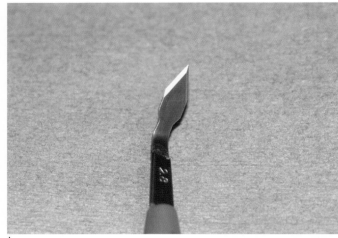

b

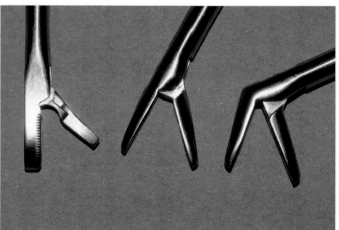

c

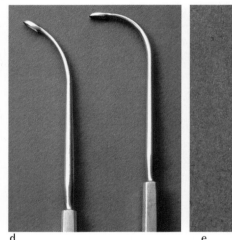

d

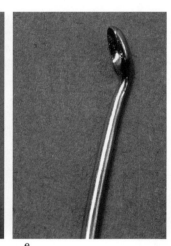

e

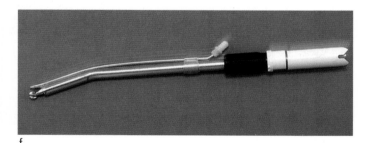

f

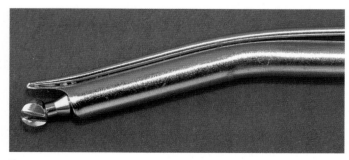

g

Figure 5.36

Endonasal instruments.
a)   Freer's elevator (centre) with straight and up-biting Blakesley forceps.
b)   2.8 mm keratome.
c)   Tips of Blakesley forceps: left, Thru-cut (has ridges); middle, straight; right, up-biting.
d)   Kuhn spoons: left, half bent; right, fully bent.
e)   J-curette.
f)   Curved straight shot drill piece.
g)   Close up of drill end.

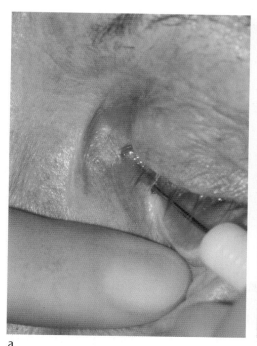

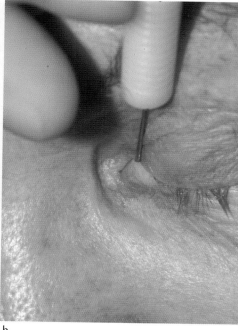

Figure 5.37

Light pipe.
a) Light pipe is inserted horizontally along the canaliculus into the lacrimal sac with the eyelid on stretch.
b) The light pipe is swung round towards the vertical, advanced then kept still.
c) The position of the light beacon is seen in the middle meatus, just posterior to the lacrimal ridge, and anterior to the uncinate process.
d) The middle turbinate is gently pushed medially using the Freer's elevator, providing a better view.

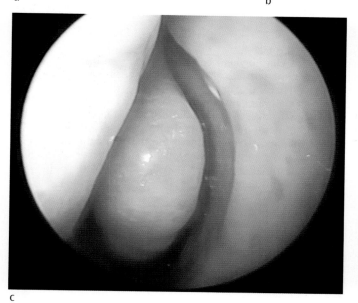

a

b

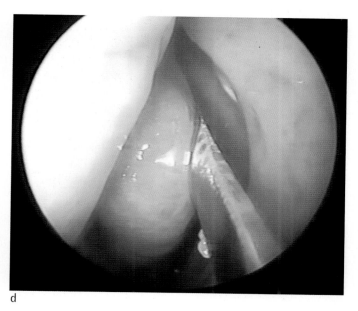

c

d

bone. NB: Do not have the light pipe turned on when inserting it, as the bright light makes it difficult to see the punctum. Some surgeons recommend only using the upper canaliculus for the light pipe (Figure 5.37).
- Inject local anaesthesia – 1 ml local anaesthetic with adrenaline (1 in 80 000) – into the lateral nasal wall at the lacrimal ridge, under direct endoscopic view.

TIP

Always introduce the second instrument (here the needle) below the endoscope (Figure 5.38).

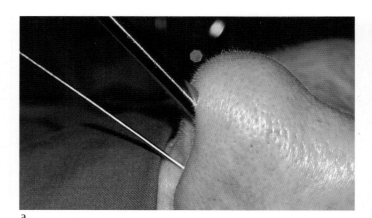

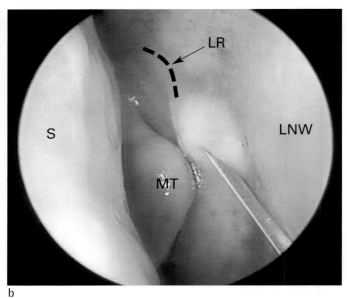

a

Figure 5.38

Local anaesthesia.
a) 4 mm diameter endoscope in nose (higher instrument) with spinal needle below.
b) Endoscopic view of left nasal space. S = septum, MT = middle turbinate, LR = lacrimal ridge, LNW = lateral nasal wall. Blanched injection bleb visible.

b

Figure 5.39

Incise nasal mucosa.
a) Freer's elevator held below endoscope, with the sharp end facing the left lateral nasal wall, prior to entering the left nasal space.
b) Freer's elevator incising the nasal mucoperiosteum at the lacrimal ridge. MT = middle turbinate, LR = lacrimal ridge.
c) Flap of nasal mucoperiosteum is raised, exposing the maxilla and lacrimal bone. Note that the light pipe beacon is clearly visible through the thin lacrimal bone. LB = lacrimal bone, MB = maxilla bone, NM = nasal mucoperiosteum.

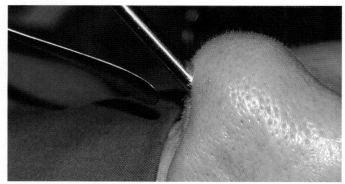

a

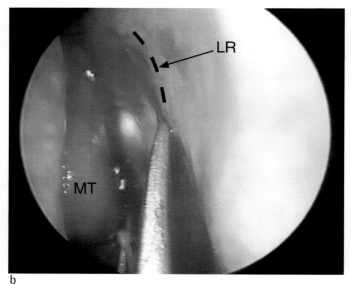

b

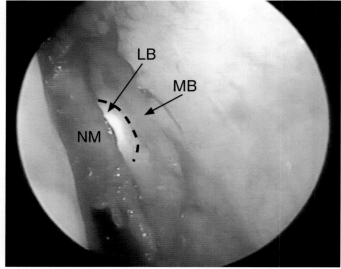

c

Incise/excise nasal mucosa

- Use the Freer's elevator to incise the nasal mucosa at or just posterior to the lacrimal ridge. Raise a flap of mucoperiosteum over the maxillary and lacrimal bone (Figure 5.39).
- Alternatively, use the J-curette or Kuhn spoon to scrape away a small area of mucoperiosteum over the lacrimal bone, from infero-posterior to antero-superior.
- Excise the flap with Blakesley forceps to reveal the underlying bone (Figure 5.40).

Remove bone

- Identify the thin lacrimal bone and the thicker maxilla bone anteriorly by moving the light pipe around or inserting a Traquair periosteal elevator and feeling the bone suture. The thin lacrimal bone is very flexible and can be pushed with the light pipe. The Traquair periosteal elevator is also useful to push the lacrimal sac mucosa laterally, away from the maxilla.
- Remove the thin lacrimal bone first, using Freer's elevator and Blakesley forceps. It often appears that there is hardly any lacrimal bone present, and it is important to seek out the small bone fragments, which could later occlude the rhinostomy.
- Kuhn spoons or the J-curette are useful to scratch and flip the thin translucent lacrimal bone off the medial aspect of the lacrimal sac. Traquair's elevator is also suitable to flip thin bone forwards (Figure 5.41).

Understanding the bony anatomy of the lateral nasal wall is *essential* for endonasal lacrimal surgery (Figure 5.42).

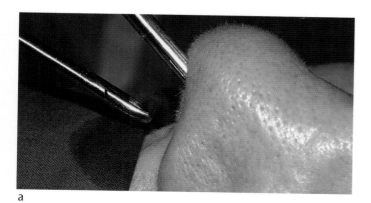

a

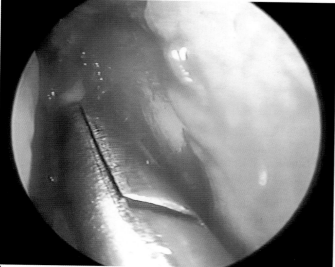

b

Figure 5.40

Excise mucoperiosteum.
a) Endoscope in nose, and straight Blakesley forceps about to enter left nasal space.
b) Straight Blakesley forceps grasping flap.
c) Bone exposed. LB = lacrimal bone, MB = maxilla bone, MT = middle turbinate. Light beacon clearly visible through thin lacrimal wall.

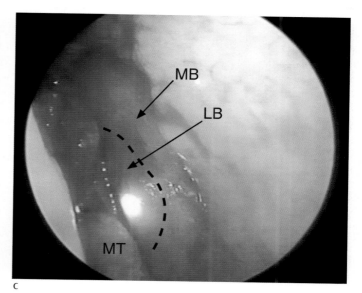

c

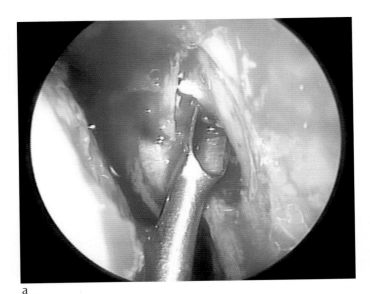

a

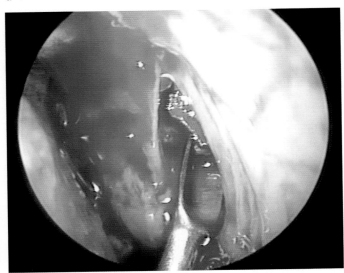

b

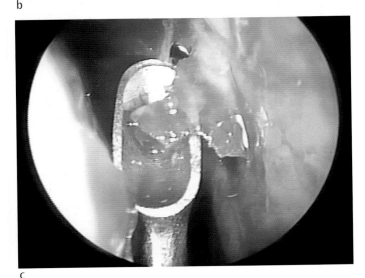

c

Figure 5.41

Remove thin lacrimal bone.
a) The light pipe elevates the lacrimal mucosa. Thin bone is detected using the J-curette.
b) The thin bone is engaged and flipped anteriorly.
c) A surprisingly large fragment of bone has been found.

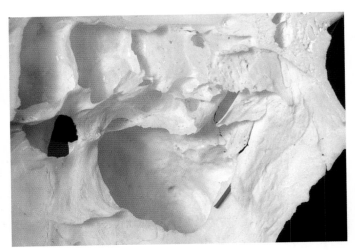

a

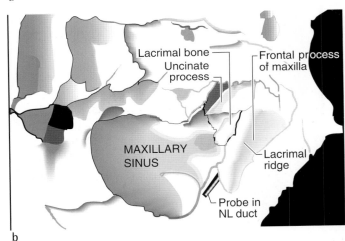

b

Figure 5.42

Endonasal bony anatomy.
a) Lateral wall of nose, showing the bones around the lacrimal sac and nasolacrimal duct. The blue probe is in the nasolacrimal canal. Note the thicker maxilla bone anteriorly, and the thin lacrimal bone posteriorly. Part of the uncinate bone is overlapping the lacrimal bone. The middle and inferior turbinates have been removed, providing a direct view into the maxillary sinus.
b) Diagram of a).

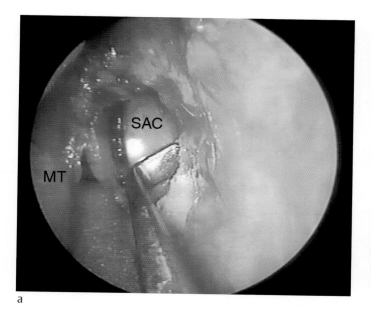
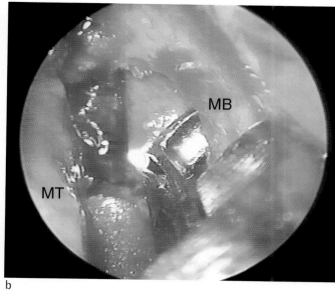

Figure 5.43

Remove thick maxilla bone.
a)   Traquair's periosteal elevator is used to feel the edge of the thick maxilla bone and push the sac mucosa laterally. Here, some maxilla has already been removed using the rongeurs. MT = middle turbinate, SAC = lacrimal sac.
b)   The Kerrison rongeur is used to take large bites of thick maxilla bone to enlarge the rhinostomy anterior to the sac. MT = middle turbinate, MB = maxilla bone.

The thin lacrimal bone is removed in a simple endonasal surgical DCR. In an extended surgical DCR, the rhinostomy is made larger and includes removal of thick maxilla bone. Some patients have a maxilla-dominant lacrimal fossa and hence require removal of thick maxilla bone (see Chapter 1). This thick maxilla bone can be removed using a hammer and chisel, forceps, or rongeurs (Figure 5.43).

Incise lacrimal sac mucosa

*   Use the light beacon to identify the sac. Move the light pipe around to determine the sac location and size, and to tent up the mucosa in order to incise its anterior surface.
*   Incise the upper part of the nasolacrimal duct and the lacrimal sac vertically, from inferior to superior, anterior to the light beacon. Do not damage the inside of the sac by pushing the blade in too deeply.

If the sac is large, additional horizontal cuts are made to produce 'flaps'. These are opened out and excess mucosa excised if necessary. Do not leave any flap of mucosa flapping, which could obstruct the common opening.

TIP

Make sure the sac incision is on the antero-medial aspect. There is a risk that if you try and incise the sac on its medial aspect the incision will be too posterior and the orbit inadvertently penetrated causing fat prolapse. By incising on the antero-medial aspect, you also have the best chance of a good view into the sac lumen (Figure 5.44).

The sucker is used during endonasal surgical DCR to aspirate blood (very little) and mucus if a mucocoele is drained (Figure 5.45). It can be used to gently pull the sac mucosa anteriorly to enable a view of the inside of the sac, and to hold the mucosa during biopsy (the specimen is not sucked up).

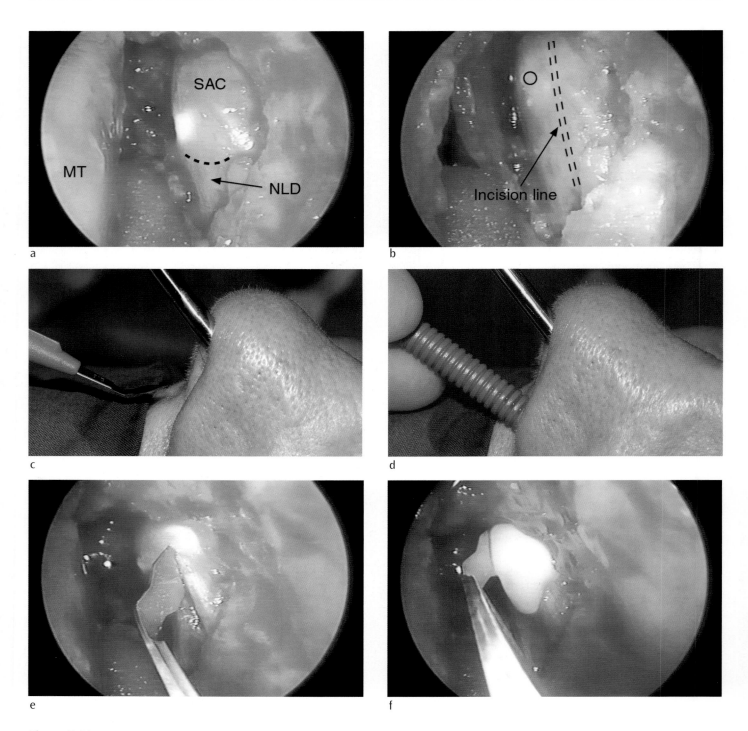

Figure 5.44

Incise the lacrimal sac and upper nasolacrimal duct mucosa.
a) The sac is identified by moving the light beacon around.
b) The incision line is anterior to the light beacon on the antero-medial aspect.
c) The keratome is inserted into the nose below the endoscope.
d) Once the keratome is inside the nose, it can be rotated under direct vision towards the sac.
e) Keratome incising mucosa from inferior to superior. The lacrimal sac is enlarged by a mucocoele.
f) Mucocoele draining internally.

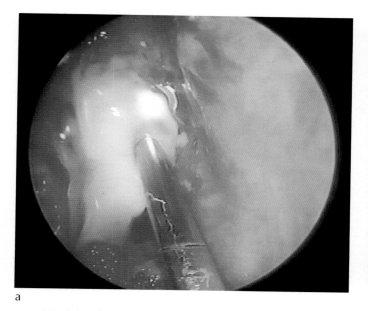

a

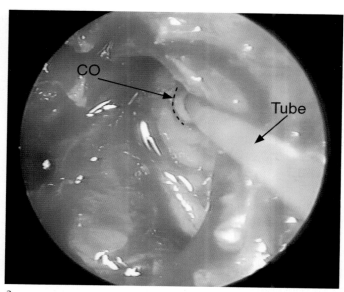

a

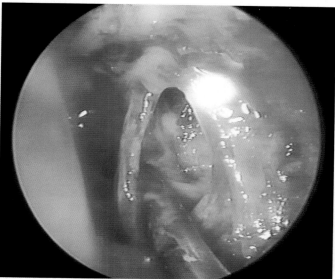

b

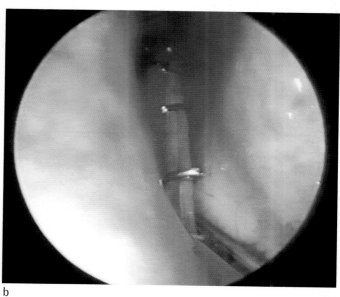

b

Figure 5.45

Sucker use.
a) The sucker is introduced into the nose, below the endoscope, under direct vision. The mucocoele is drained and mucus/debris aspirated.
b) The inside of the sac is cleaned gently, and any early dacryoliths removed. In this sac there was a thick plaque of inspissated mucus lining the medial wall. The inside of the sac is seen. The mucosal lining is oedematous and inflamed.

Figure 5.46

Intubation.
a) The bodkin emerging from the common opening has been grasped by an artery clip and the tube pulled through. The common opening (CO) is seen.
b) Both tubes are in place. These tubes have been secured with Ligaclips. Knots are equally effective and are cheaper.

Pass and secure O'Donoghue tubes

Temporary silicone tube intubation is usual. Short bodkined tubes (30 mm blunt bodkin with 40 cm silicone tube) are recommended.

- Bend the bodkins slightly and insert one via the canaliculus used for the light pipe. After reaching the sac, rotate the bodkin downwards and slightly medially, with the bodkin curve convex anteriorly in order to present the tip within the middle meatus. Take care not to touch the middle turbinate or septum and damage the mucosa.
- Use a curved artery clip to grasp the tip of the bodkin and pull the tube through into the nose.
- Repeat via the second canaliculus.
- Cut the bodkins off and tie the tubes with six to eight knots, or secure the ends with four titanium Ligaclips, or use a combination of both.
- Check the position of the uppermost knot or clip without the tubes on tension; it should be approximately 3–5 mm below the rhinostomy to allow for healing and tube movement on blinking (Figure 5.46).

TIP
When passing the tubes the artery clip grasps the bodkin tip, which prevents the tip damaging the floor or vestibule when pulling the bodkins out of the nose.

ii) Endonasal laser DCR

There are two endonasal lasers commonly used for DCR; holmium : YAG and KTP : NdYAG. Surgery is either entirely by laser ablation or is combined with endosurgical techniques – for instance, removing thicker bone surgically and using the keratome to incise the lacrimal mucosa. Combining laser and surgical techniques gives better results than using the laser alone. Adjuvant anti-metabolite mitomycin C may improve results although there are reservations about its use – see Figure 5.66.

Other lasers: Originally (1990) a high-powered argon laser (16 W) was used, which is well absorbed by melanin and haemaglobin; it is therefore adequate for mucosa but not for bone. The CO_2 laser was tried, but delivery was difficult.

The holmium : YAG laser

This is a 2100 nm pulsed laser. It works very well in water, which it heats and vaporizes, and has to be held close to the target tissue. It has a 0.4 mm penetration depth, and therefore is regarded as relatively safe for endonasal DCR.

The KTP : NdYAG laser

KTP = potassium titanyl phosphate. This is a 532 nm super-pulsed, frequency-doubled laser, which is good for mucosa and bone ablation. Powers of up to 15 W are used in near-contact mode, using a fine 300 μm or 400 μm fibre. Tissue penetration is up to 4 mm, which is

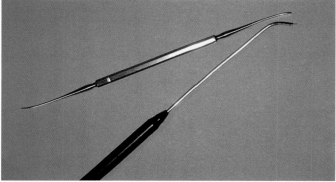

a

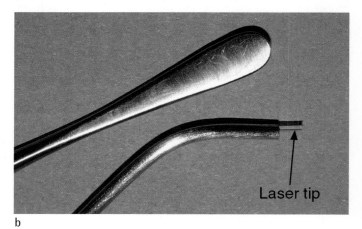

Laser tip

b

Figure 5.47

Endonasal laser.
a)   Angled holmium : YAG laser probe and Freer's elevator.
b)   Close up of laser tip and elevator.

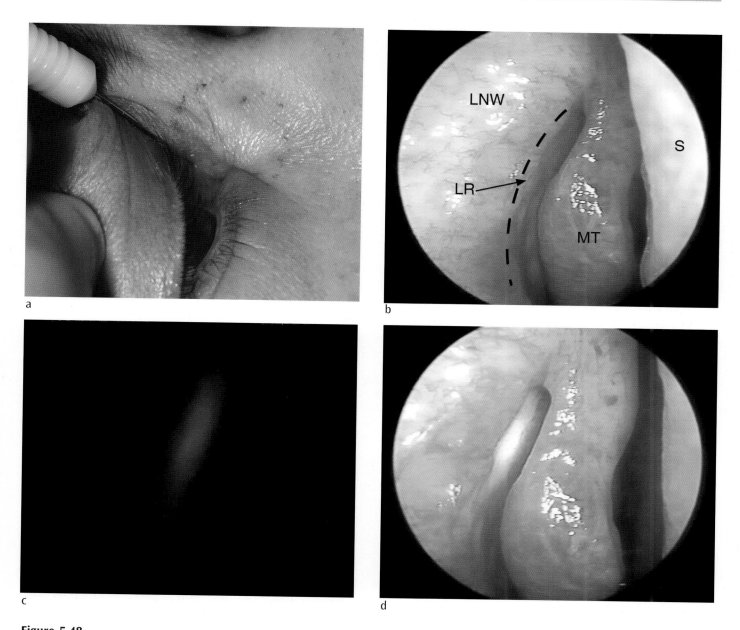

Figure 5.48

Light pipe beacon identified endonasally.
a)   The light pipe is correctly placed.
b)   The middle turbinate (MT) and lacrimal ridge (LR) are identified on the lateral nasal wall (LNW). S = septum.
c)   Once the light pipe is turned on it should be visible on the lateral nasal wall. Reducing or turning off the endoscope light helps in locating the light beacon.
d)   The light beacon is seen just posterior to the lacrimal ridge below the neck of the middle turbinate.

excellent for bone ablation but potentially dangerous within the lacrimal sac. The Laserscope® KTP laser penetrates 0.3–0.5 mm using star pulse, and 1 mm using continous mode. KTP has excellent haemostatic properties, but can cause tissue char and some adjacent mucosal damage. Protective goggles must be worn to protect theatre personnel from the green visible light along the fibres, and a special filter placed in the endoscope head, in front of the camera, to protect it from burning out.

Sucker

Whichever laser is used, the smoke produced from the tissue ablation must be extracted using a sucker placed in the nose.

Holmium : YAG laser settings:
- Fibre diameter 300, 400 or 500 μm
- Mucosa – 0.6 or 0.8 J at 10 Hz, i.e. 6–8 W
- Bone – 1.0 J at 10 Hz, i.e. 10 W.

KTP : NdYAG laser settings (Lasercope®):
- Fibre diameter 400 μm
- Mucosa 50–60 W star pulse for 10 ms pulse widths, 20 pulses per second = 5 W
- Bone – 60–70 W star pulse for 5 ms pulse widths, 20 pulses per second = 6–7 W
- Thick bone – continuous wave for 7–15 W.

Instruments for endolaser surgery (Figure 5.48):
These are very simple, and include:
- Laser handle and fibre
- Freer's elevator
- Sucker
- Nettleship dilator
- Light pipe.

The surgical steps are similar to endonasal surgical DCR. The laser can be used to ablate the nasal mucosa, intervening bone and lacrimal sac mucosa.

Insert light pipe and inject nasal anaesthesia

Inserting the light pipe and injecting local anaesthesia is similar to endonasal surgical DCR. In endonasal laser DCR there may be bleeding from the local injection (Figure 5.48).

Ablate nasal mucosa, bone and lacrimal sac mucosa

Displace the middle turbinate medially with Freer's elevator as necessary – e.g. with a paradoxically curved turbinate or concha bullosa (Figure 5.49). The laser

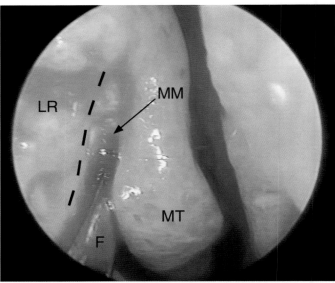

a

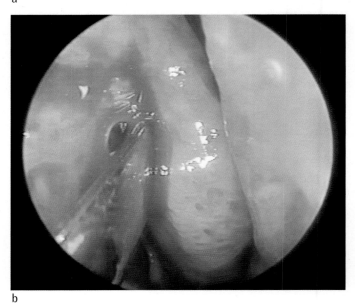

b

Figure 5.49

Displace middle turbinate.
a)   Freer's elevator (F) is placed in the middle meatus (MM), where there is a middle turbinate (MT) variation (paradoxical curvature). The light beacon is posterior to the lacrimal ridge (LR) shown by the dotted line. The bleeding is from the local anaesthesia injection.
b)   The middle turbinate is pushed medially, away from the middle meatus.

ablates the mucosa and thin lacrimal bone and enters the lacrimal sac. The final rhinostomy measures 4–6 mm. Some surgeons recommend opening the

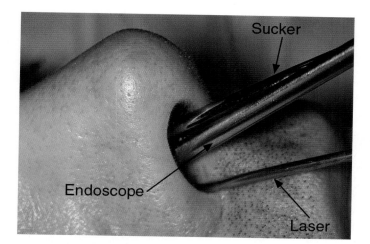

Figure 5.50

Endonasal laser DCR requires three instruments in the nose. The laser probe and sucker are inserted below the endoscope.

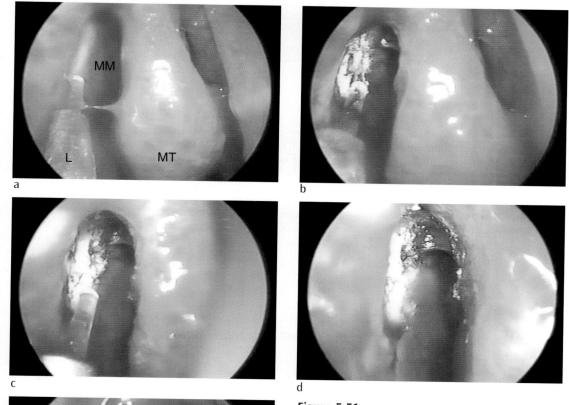

Figure 5.51

Holmium : YAG laser.
a) The laser (L) is held close to the target site (light beacon) in the middle meatus (MM). The middle turbinate (MT) remains untouched.
b) The mucosa is ablated and the smoke evacuated. During surgery the endoscope is held anterior to the laser to avoid blur from tissue splutter and reduce the need to remove the endoscope for cleaning.
c) Increased nasal mucosal and thin lacrimal bone ablation. A small amount of collateral mucosal damage is visible at the neck of the middle turbinate, which might become a small synaechiae later.
d) The bright light beacon is visible over an area approximately 4–5 mm in diameter.
e) A mucocoele drains. LNW = lateral nasal wall, MT = middle turbinate.

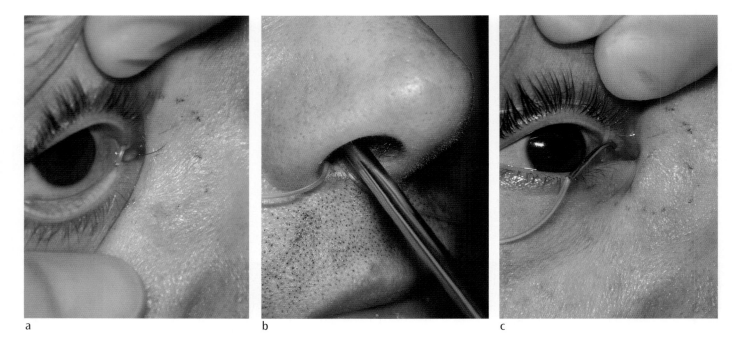

a   b   c

Figure 5.52

Intubation.
a) Curve the bodkin and gently pass it down into the sac, through the ostium and into the nose. In order to pass the bodkin into the nose, its convexity is kept *anterior*. If any resistance is felt, do not push; this can damage the mucosa. Instead, check that the canaliculus is on stretch and that the tip has entered the sac and is not kinking the canaliculus. It should pass easily into the nose; if not, the rhinostomy needs enlarging.
b) Once the bodkins are detached and the tubes knotted, the endoscope is used to check the position of the knots in relation to the surgical rhinostomy. The ends are then trimmed, to lie at the level of the inferior turbinate.
c) When checking the intranasal position of the tubes, simultaneously check that there is normal tube tension at the medial canthus, to avoid the complication of punctual cheesewiring.

lacrimal sac mucosa with a shallow-tipped blade rather than laser to reduce the risk of intra-sac damage, in particular the common opening (Figures 5.50, 5.51).

Pass tubes

This is similar to endonasal surgical DCR. Pass the tubes into the nose, where they are knotted or clipped to secure them. NB: Take great care to avoid mucosal damage at the middle meatus or floor when catching the bodkin tip with a curved artery clip (Figure 5.52).

Use of anti-metabolites after endosurgical or endolaser DCR

The use of a single per-operative application of mitomycin C to reduce or eliminate post-operative scarring is still controversial, and it has not been in use for long enough to assess the long-term sequelae fully. There is a risk of delayed nasal mucosal healing leaving bare bone, which theoretically predisposes to infection. In the future, precise application to a small area may be identified where there are risk factors.

Part C: Post-operative management

Post-operative management is divided into early, intermediate and late.

Early management

At the end of surgery

External DCR:
- Padding the eye/wound is optional
- Sit the patient up at 45° as soon as possible to reduce bleeding
- Avoid nose-blowing for 4–7 days
- Prescribe broad-spectrum systemic antibiotics for 1 week, or give an antibiotic bolus per-operatively if a mucocoele or sinusitis is noted
- Give topical steroid and antibiotic eyedrops for 3 weeks.

Endonasal DCR:
- There is usually no nasal pack
- Sit patient up as for external DCR
- Avoid nose-blowing for 4–7 days
- Give topical steroid and antibiotic eyedrops for 4 weeks
- There is usually no need for nasal steroid spray.

> Practice point: Post-operative instructions to the patient must be clear – e.g. avoid blowing nose for up to 1 week, to prevent nasal haemorrhage and orbital emphysema.

Outpatients follow-up

External DCR: 1 week for removal of sutures; between 1 and 3 months for removal of tubes; and 6 months after surgery for the last check. Follow-up is more frequent if there are complications.

Endonasal DCR: 1 or 2 weeks to check nose and position of tubes; between 2 and 3 months for removal of tubes; and 6 months after surgery for the last check. Follow-up is more frequent if there are complications.

At the 1 or 2 week post-operative visit

- Reassure the patient if there is still some watering, which may be due to the presence of the tubes or

the persistence of crusting within the surgical rhinostomy.

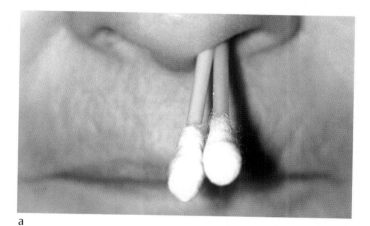

a

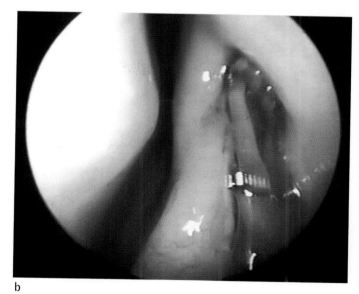

b

Figure 5.53

a) Cotton buds with guttae phenylephrine placed in nasal space for mucosal decongestion.
b) Appearance of left surgical ostium 1 week after external DCR and tubes (one flap only). Healing is not quite complete. There is a Watzke sleeve high up in the rhinostomy, which may be a problem later. A Ligaclip is below the ostium.

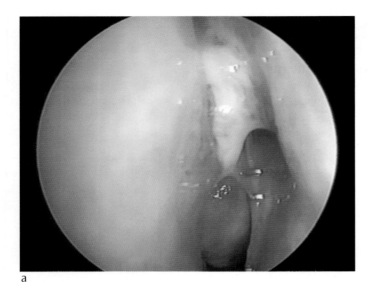

a

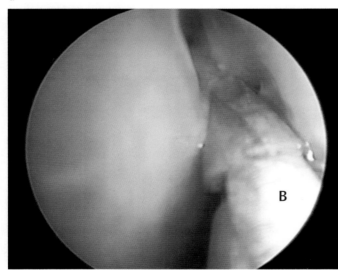

B

b

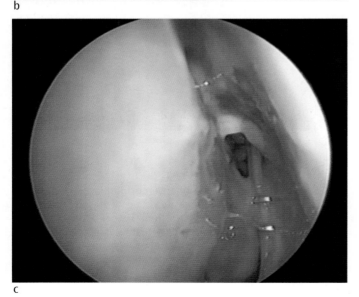

c

Figure 5.54

Left nasal space 1 week after endonasal surgical DCR.
a) There is an early soft synaechia present anterior to the rhinostomy, between the septum (left) and lateral nasal wall (right). The tubes are visible behind, and fluorescein confirms free passage of dye from the conjunctival sac into the nose.
b) Straight Blakesley forceps are used to grasp and remove the synaechiae. B = Blakesley forceps.
c) Appearance after treatment. There is a better view of the surgical rhinostomy.

- Encourage the patient to start to blow the nose in order to clear out old blood clots and crusts. If external DCR was performed, inspect the external wound for dehiscence or infection.
- Remove the skin sutures.
- Examine the nasal space after decongestion with guttae phenylephrine 2.5% or 10% on cotton buds, or co-phenylcaine nasal spray. Inspect tube movement on blinking, and their position in relation to the rhinostomy. Remove crusts with forceps as necessary, and divide early synaechiae when needed. Start broad-spectrum antibiotics if excessive mucous discharge is seen across the rhinostomy from chronic rhinosinus disease.

By 1 week, the mucosal healing should be almost complete for external DCR and still incomplete for endonasal DCR (Figure 5.53).

Early synaechiae between the lateral nasal wall and septum, or between the middle turbinate and lateral nasal wall, are easily divided and removed whilst they are soft, 1 week after surgery (Figure 5.54).

Crusts lying within the rhinostomy are removed with Blakesley forceps (Figure 5.55).

Crusts can be annoying to the patient and extra visits may be required (Figure 5.56).

Intermediate management (up to 3 months)

- Plan removal of the tubes 2–12 weeks after surgery, depending on the indication for their placement.

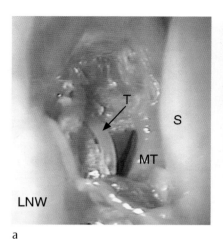

a

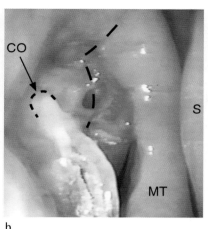

b

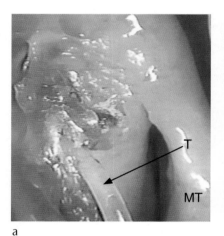

a

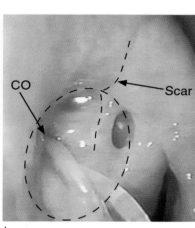

b

Figure 5.55

Right surgical rhinostomy one week after re-do external DCR and tubes with one sutured anterior flap (posterior flap not sutured).
a) Crusts are lying within the rhinostomy and surrounding the tubes (T), which are emerging from the common canaliculus on the lateral nasal wall (LNW) close to the anterior end of the neck of the middle turbinate (MT). The septum (S) is on the right.
b) The crusts are removed by Blakesley forceps. The lacrimal sac mucosa is now visible, with the tubes emerging from the common canalicular (CC) opening. The line of incomplete posterior mucosal healing (secondary intention) is visible. MT = middle turbinate, S = septum.

Figure 5.56

Three weeks after surgery (same patient as Figure 5.55).
a) Persistent crusts in rhinostomy. T = tubes, MT = middle turbinate. The crusts are again removed with Blakesley forceps.
b) Clean healed rhinostomy. The shallow depression formed by the healed rhinostomy in the lateral nasal wall and the posterior scar are outlined. There is a small opening into the sinus. The tubes emerge from the common opening (CO).

- Before cutting the tubes at the medial canthus, inspect the nasal space endoscopically to detect pathology, and inspect the healed rhinostomy and tubes. Nasal mucosal vasoconstriction is recommended, but topical anaesthesia is not usually required, either on the eye or in the nose.
- Cut the tubes at the medial canthus, and then either ask the patient to lean forward and blow the nose to blow the tubes out, or to gently retrieve them under direct endoscopic visualization. This is atraumatic and quick (Figure 5.57).
- After the tubes are removed, syringe the lacrimal system to wash through any mucus and confirm patency.

- Perform a functional endoscopic dye test, and inspect the healed rhinostomy (Figure 5.58).

Late management (6 months after surgery)

Evaluate the success of surgery.
1. Subjective results:
   - Ask if the epiphora and stickiness has improved or been cured. The patient should estimate how much improvement there is (100 per cent maximum) compared to before the surgery.

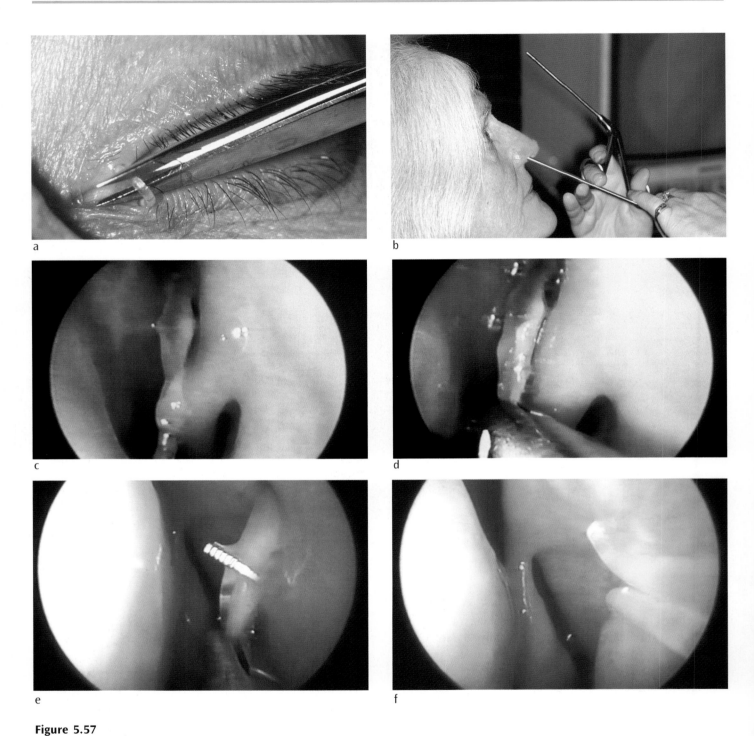

Figure 5.57

Endoscopic endonasal removal of tubes.
a)   After the tubes are located endonasally, they are divided at the medial canthus.
b)   The patient sits, and the tubes are retrieved under direct endoscopic visualization.
c)   The tubes ends are seen at the level of the inferior turbinate (left side).
d)   The tubes are grasped with Blakesley forceps at the level of the inferior meatus under direct view and retrieved from the nose.
e)   These tubes are grasped higher up, above the inferior turbinate, close to the surgical rhinostomy (left side).
f)   The tubes are removed.

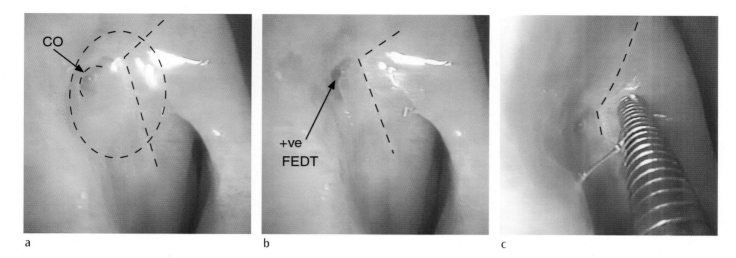

a   b   c

Figure 5.58

Healed rhinostomy (same patient as in Figures 5.55, 5.56).
a) Appearance after removal of tubes 8 weeks after re-do external DCR. Common opening (CO). The edge of the healed rhinostomy and posterior flap scar are outlined.
b) Dye placed in the conjunctival sac rapidly emerges from the common opening and drains down the lateral nasal wall. This is a positive functional endoscopic dye test (+ve FEDT).
c) A measure has been placed adjacent to the rhinostomy. Each graduation measures 0.5 mm. The rhinostomy forms a shallow alcove in the lateral nasal wall, approximately 8 mm in diameter. The central common canalicular opening is approximately 2–2.5 mm in diameter.

2. Objective results:
    • Syringe the lacrimal system.
    • Do a final endonasal examination to observe the functional endoscopic dye test.

Anatomical and functional success is defined as improvement of symptoms, patent syringing and a positive FEDT. Some patients with previous nasolacrimal duct obstruction have improvement of symptoms and patent syringing but a negative FEDT; they exhibit an alternative drainage route, probably via the ethmoid or maxilla sinus.

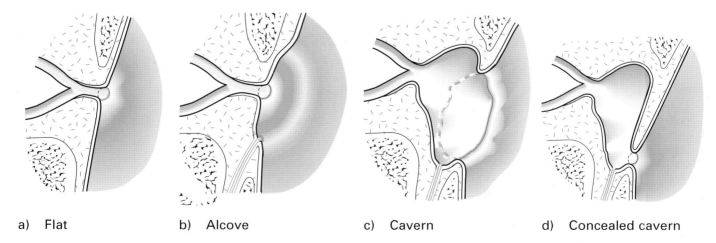

a) Flat   b) Alcove   c) Cavern   d) Concealed cavern

Figure 5.59

Rhinostomy variations on lateral nasal wall.

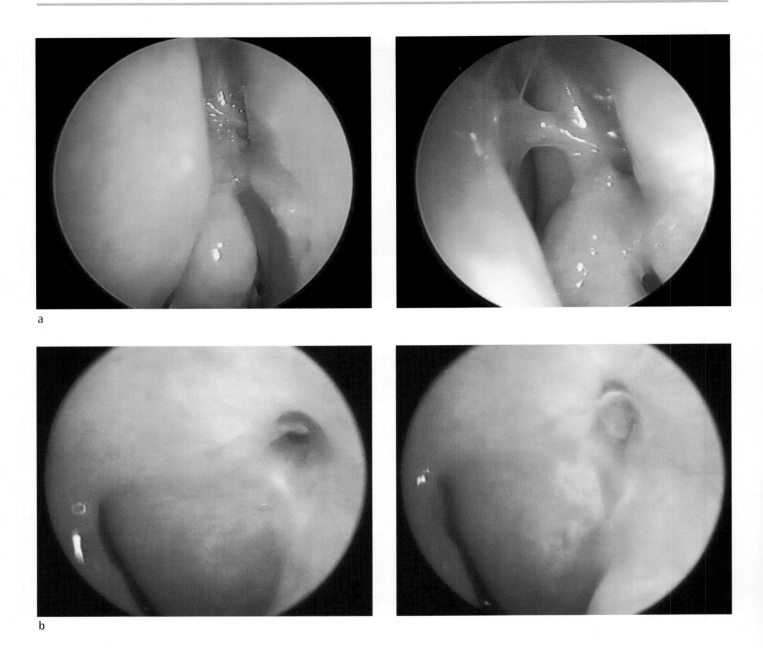

a

b

Figure 5.60

Healed DCR rhinostomies.
a)   Left: Appearance 6 months after left endonasal surgical DCR. There are fine synaechiae between the posterior edge of the rhinostomy and the septum, which do not interfere with function.
     Right: Positive FEDT.
b)   Left: Appearance 6 months after left external DCR. Round cavernous ostium, more anterior than above.
     Right: Positive FEDT.

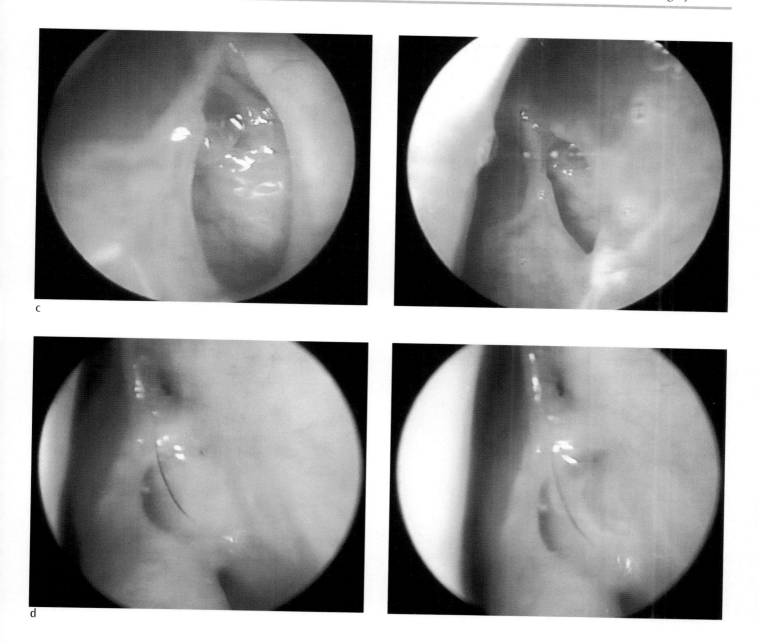

Figure 5.60 *continued*

Healed DCR rhinostomies.
c)   Left: Appearance 6 months after left endosurgical DCR. Deep alcove/shallow cavern. Note the common opening in the upper part and the early phase of a positive FEDT.
Right: Same rhinostomy, lower magnification, with fluorescein draining down the lateral nasal wall.
d)   Left: Appearance 6 months after left external DCR. There is a flat profiled rhinostomy with a small opening visible, probably the common canaliculus.
Right: Same rhinostomy, positive FEDT. The opening above has no fluorescein and is probably into the ethmoid.

Healed rhinostomy appearance

The appearance of the rhinostomy varies greatly between patients and depends on the original size and location of the rhinostomy, the thickness of intervening bone and the condition of the mucosa, as well as the type of DCR done. A functioning rhinostomy can be flat or cavernous. There is no apparent difference between the size and appearance of the healed rhinostomy after external DCR compared to endonasal surgical DCR, but the healed rhinostomy after endolaser DCR appears smaller (Figures 5.59, 5.60).

Complications after DCR

Early complications – 1–4 weeks:
- Wound infection, fistula or dehiscence
- Tube lateral displacement
- Medial corneal erosion from tubes at medial canthus
- Excessive rhinostomy crusting
- Intranasal synaechiae
- Delayed healing secondary to application of anti-metabolites, e.g. mitomycin C.

Intermediate complications – 1–3 months:
- Intranasal synaechiae
- Rhinostomy fibrosis

- Granulomas at rhinostomy
- Tube lateral displacement
- Corneal erosion from tubes
- Punctal cheesewiring
- Punctal/canalicular pyogenic granuloma
- Tube tie impaction in ostium
- Prominent facial scar
- Medial canthal distortion
- Persistent fistula to skin from recurrent dacryocystitis in non-functioning DCR.

Late complications – 6 months:
- Rhinostomy fibrosis
- Delayed mucosal healing (anti-metabolite)
- Persistent intranasal synaechiae
- Webbed facial scar (external DCR)
- Medial canthal distortion
- Chronic fistula (non-functioning DCR).

Tube prolapse or lateral displacement

This is rare (occurs in less than 3 per cent of patients). It occurs 1–4 weeks after surgery. Predisposing factors include lower eyelid laxity, loss of tie or a low tie on the tubes, and a cavernous rhinostomy. The patient catches the tube at the medial canthus with a finger and pulls it partially out.

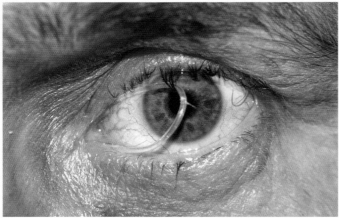

a

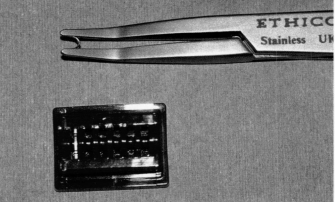

b

Figure 5.61

Tube displacement.
a)   Left lateral displacement tubes.
b)   Ligaclip and applicator.

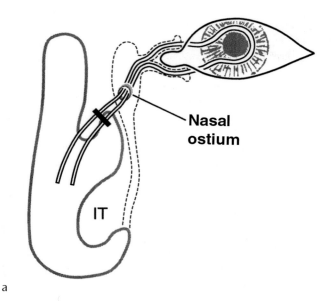

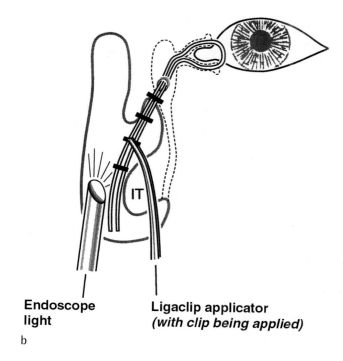

Figure 5.62

Diagram showing a), displaced tube, and b), endoscopic repositioning under topical anaesthesia.

Displaced tubes can be pushed back in from above or pulled down inside the nose, using either an indirect ophthalmoscope as the light source or an endoscope. If the tie is low and there is a risk of recurrent prolapse, the tubes are further secured with Ligaclips above the existing tie under direct endoscopic view (Figures 5.61, 5.62).

Synaechiae and granulomata

Transnasal synaechiae and granulomata may obstruct the rhinostomy (Figure 5.63). If detected in the early post-operative phase, they can sometimes be treated.

Granulomata are treated using a silver nitrate stick or excision. If the granuloma is peri-rhinostomy, it is likely that the surgery will fail; if it is para-rhinostomy, the opening may be kept patent (Figure 5.64).

Delayed nasal mucosal healing following mitomycin C application at surgery

Mitomycin C (MMC) is advocated by some surgeons to reduce scarring and hence improve success. However,

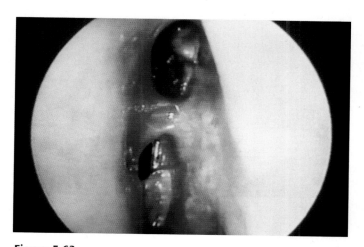

Figure 5.63

Left extensive transnasal synaechiae and ostium granuloma. The tubes were immobile on blinking and the ostium non-functional after the removal of tubes.

great care must be taken in MMC application at surgery and only the lowest doses used, as the anti-metabolite can permanently affect tissue healing (Figure 5.65).

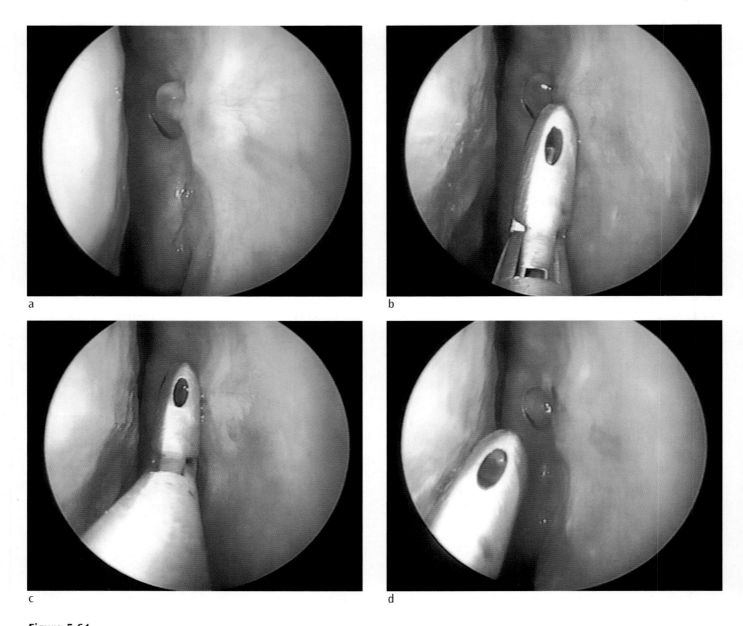

a

b

c

d

Figure 5.64

Granuloma snaring.
a) Small granuloma anterior to ostium (para-ostium), left nasal space.
b) Up-biting Blakesley forceps introduced into nasal space.
c) Granuloma grasped.
d) Granuloma removed.

Punctal cheesewiring

If the tubes are tied too tightly in the nose, they risk cheesewiring the lower punctum (Figure 5.67).

Facial disfigurement

Rarely, external approach DCR results in a webbed medial canthal scar or medial canthal displacement. The

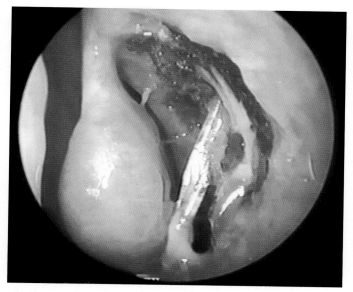

Figure 5.65

Appearance of left rhinostomy 4 weeks after endonasal holmium laser DCR with application of mitomycin C 0.2 mg/ml for 3 minutes. Note the bare bone anterior to the rhinostomy.

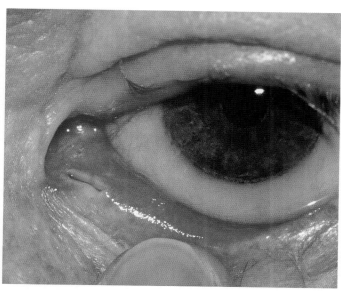

Figure 5.66

Left lower punctal/canalicular cheesewiring.

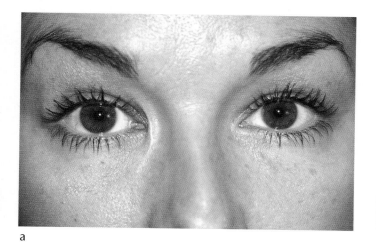

a

Figure 5.67

Scar revision.
a) Right webbed scar 1 year after right external DCR.
b) Side view.

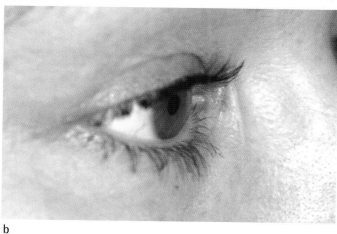

b

continued overleaf

surgeon has probably placed the incision too close to the medial canthal angle, or damaged the underlying orbicularis muscle or medial canthal tendon. In the first 6 months after surgery, reassure the patient and advise that the prominent or webbed scar should be massaged with moisturizing cream (with factor 15 sun-screen). Wait at least 1 year before considering scar revision (Figure 5.67).

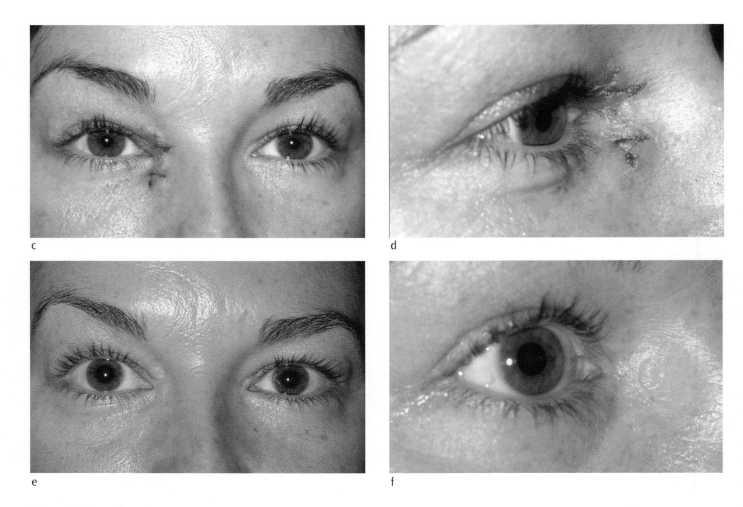

c
d
e
f

Figure 5.67 *continued*

Scar revision.
c)   Double Z plasty and excision of scar (flaps are positioned for suturing).
d)   Side view of same.
e)   Result 6 months after scar revision.
f)   Side view of same.

Bibliography

Boush, G. A., Lempke, B. N. and Dortzbach, R. K. (1994). Results of endonasal laser-assisted dacryocystorhinostomy. *Ophthalmology.*, 101, 955–9.

Caldwell, G. W. (1893). Two new operations for obstruction of the nasolacrimal duct with preservation of the canaliculi, and an incidental description of a new lacrimal probe. *NY Med. J.*, 57, 581.

Camera, J. G., Benzon, A. U. and Henson, R. D. (2000). The safety and efficacy of mitomycin C in endonasal endoscopic laser assisted dacryocystorhinostomy. *Ophthal. Plast. Reconstr. Surg.*, 16, 114–18.

Dupuy-Dutemps, and Bourguet. (1921). Procede plastique de dacryocysto-rhinostomie et ses resultats. *Annales d'Oculistique*, 158, 241–61.

Hallam, A. V. (1949). The Dupuy-Dutemps dacryocystorhinostomy. *Am. J. Ophthalmol.*, 32, 1197–1206.

Harris, G. J., Sakol, P. J. and Beatty, R. L. (1989). Relaxed skin tension line incision for dacryocystorhinostomy. *Am. J. Ophthalmol.*, 108, 742–3.

Jokinen, K. and Kerja, J. (1974). Endonasal dacryocystorhinostomy. *Arch. Otolaryngol. Head Neck Surg.*, 100, 41–4.

Jones, L. T. and Boyden, G. L. (1951). The rhinologist's role in tear sac surgery. *Trans. Am. Acad. Ophth. Otol.*, Jul–Aug, 654–61.

Jones, L. T. and Boyden, G. L. (1962). New mucous membrane flap for dacryocystorhinostomy. *AMA Arch. Otolaryngol.*, 405–8.

Linberg, J. V., Anderson, R. L. L., Bumstead, R. M. and Barreras, R. (1982). Study of intranasal osteum external dacryocystorhinostomy. *Arch. Ophthalmol.*, 100, 1758–62.

Massaro, B., Gonnering, R. and Harris, G. (1990). Endonasal laser dacryocystorhinostomy. *Arch. Ophthalmol.*, 108, 1172–6.

McDonough, M. and Meiring, J. H. (1989). Endoscopic transnasal dacryocystorhinostomy. *J. Laryngol. Otol.*, 103, 585–7.

Metson, R. (1991). Endoscopic surgery for lacrimal obstruction. *Otolaryngol. Head Neck Surg.*, 104, 473–9.

Minasian, M. and Olver, J. M. (1999). The value of nasal endoscopy after dacryocystorhinostomy. *Orbit.*, 18, 167–76.

Olver, J. M. and Minasian, M. (1998). Nasal endoscopy for ophthalmologists. *CME J. Ophthalmol.*, 2, 73–7.

Orcutt, J. C., Hillel, A. and Weymuller, E. A. (1990). Endoscopic repair of failed dacryocystorhinostomy. *Ophthal. Plast. Reconstr. Surg.*, 6, 197–202.

Quickert, M.H. and Dryden, R.M. (1970). Probes for intubation in lacrimal drainage. *Trans. Am. Acad. Ophthalmol. Otolaryngol.*, 74(2); 431–3.

Sadiq, S. A., Hugkulstone, C. E., Jones, N. S. and Downes, R. N. (1996). Endoscopic holmium : YAG laser dacryocystorhinostomy. *Eye.*, 10, 43–6.

Steadman, G. M. (1985). Transnasal dacryocystorhinostomy. *Otolaryngol. Clin. North Am.*, 18, 107–11.

Szubin, L., Papageoreg, A. and Sacks, E. (1999). Endonasal laser assisted dacryocystorhinostomy. *Am. J. Rhinol.*, 13, 371–4.

Toti, A. (1904). Nuovo metodo conservatore di cura radicale delle suppurazione croniche del saco lacrimale (dacriocisto rinostomia). *La Clinica Moderna*, 10, 385–7.

Wearne, M. J., Beigi, B., Davis, G. and Rose, G. E. (1999). Retrograde intubation dacryocystorhinostomy for proximal and midcanalicular obstruction. *Ophthalmology.*, 106, 2325–9.

Welham, R. A. N. and Henderson, P. H. (1973). Results of dacryocystorhinostomy: analysis of causes of failure. *Trans. Ophthalmol. Soc. UK.*, 93, 601–9.

West, J. M. (1914). A window resection in the nasal duct in cases of stenosis. *Trans. Am. Ophthalmol. Soc.*, 12, 654–8.

Whittet, H. B., Shun-Shin, G. A. and Awdry, P. (1993). Functional endoscopic transnasal dacryocystorhinostomy. *Eye.*, 7, 545–9.

Woog, J. J., Metson, R. and Puliafito, C. A. (1993). Holmium : YAG endonasal laser dacryocystorhinostomy. *Am. J. Ophthalmol.*, 116, 1–10.

Yung, M. W. and Hardman-Lea, S. (1998). Endoscopic inferior dacryocystorhinostomy. *Clin. Otolaryngol.*, 23, 152–7.

Zilelioglu, G., Ugurbas, S. H., Anadolu, Y. *et al.* (1998). Adjunctive use of mitomycin C on endoscopic lacrimal surgery. *Br. J. Ophthalmol.*, 82, 63–6.

CHAPTER 6

Canalicular Surgery

In this chapter the management of acquired punctal and canalicular problems, such as actinomycoses canaliculitis, canalicular trauma and longstanding canalicular obstruction, are described.

The chapter is divided as follows:

Part A: Localized punctal and proximal canalicular problems

Part B: Acute canalicular trauma

Part C: Longstanding canalicular obstructions.

Part A: Localized punctal and proximal canalicular problems

Acquired punctal stenosis

Age or inflammation causes a fibrous ring around the punctum. Ectropion causes a dry, stenosed, non-functioning punctum. Exclude all other possible causes of epiphora before considering lower punctoplasty or canaliculoplasty.

Management

1. *Punctoplasty.* Dilate the punctum well with a Nettleship dilator. If there is a membrane, spin down vertically onto it with an orange needle (size 25).
2. *Canaliculoplasty.* Enlarge punctum by one or three snips (Figure 6.1).

One-snip procedure

This opens the vertical part of the punctum into the ampulla on the posterior aspect of the lower lid. It is *not* an elegant procedure, and often closes off again.

● Dilate the lower punctum with a Nettleship dilator, keeping the eyelid on lateral stretch
● Cut down onto the dilator on the posterior aspect of the eyelid using a fine blade, or insert straight, sharp scissors almost vertically with the Nettleship dilator removed.

Three-snip procedure

This fully opens the ampulla and proximal part of the canaliculus on the posterior aspect of the lower lid. The three-snip procedure can permanently damage the proximal canaliculus, and is not always effective.

● Dilate the punctum well and extend the dilator along the proximal canaliculus (up to 4 mm), with the lower eyelid on lateral stretch
● Cut down on the posterior aspect or use scissors as for the one snip

● Open less than one-third of the length of the canaliculus using the blade or scissors
● Remove a small posterior lamella triangle of posterior conjunctiva and canaliculus.

Papillomatosis at medial canthus

Papillomatosis (Figure 6.2) arises most commonly from the inferior retropunctal or medial tarsal/plical

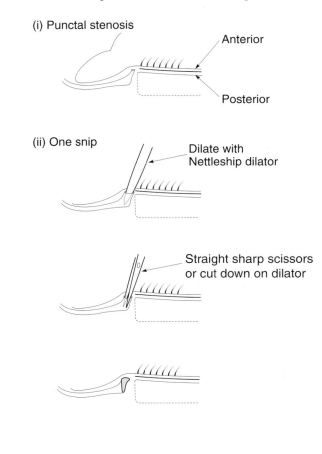

Figure 6.1

One- and three-snip canaliculoplasty for punctal stenosis.

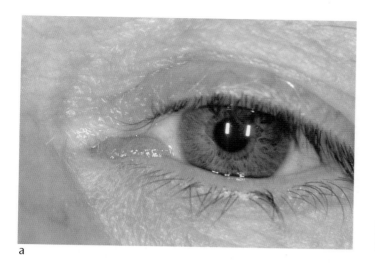

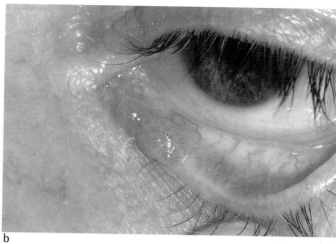

Figure 6.2

Medial canthal papilloma arising from the tarsal conjunctiva, occluding the punctum.

conjunctiva, and rarely from the canaliculus or punctum. It is unilateral, of viral origin, and has a tendency to recur. It causes mild obstructive epiphora and a visible mass.

Management

Management is by local excision.

- Identify the punctum and place a Bowman probe size 0 in the canaliculus
- Find the papilloma base and excise it completely
- Diathermy the base thoroughly to ensure that all papilloma tissue is destroyed
- If the papilloma is in the punctum or canaliculus, use adjunctive cryotherapy
- Perform canaliculoplasty if the papilloma is within the canaliculus – if in doubt, open the ampulla and inspect the mucosal lining.

Granuloma at medial canthus

This appears as a pinkish inflammatory mass around silicone tubes or a glass bypass tube.

Management

1. Silicone tubes *in situ*:
   - Remove tubes and diathermy the granuloma at its base
   - Apply topical steroid drops.
2. Glass Jones bypass tube left in:
   - Leave tube in if possible
   - Locally excise the granuloma
   - Apply light silver nitrate treatment to its base
   - Apply topical steroid drops (see Figure 6.3).

Actinomycoses canaliculitis

This is also called streptothrix. Actinomycoses is a facultative anaerobe or strict anaerobic gram-positive bacillus, usually arranged in hyphae although it can fragment into short bacilli. It is a mouth commensal. True fungal organisms can also cause canaliculitis. Both acute and chronic canaliculitis are easily missed (see Figure 6.4).

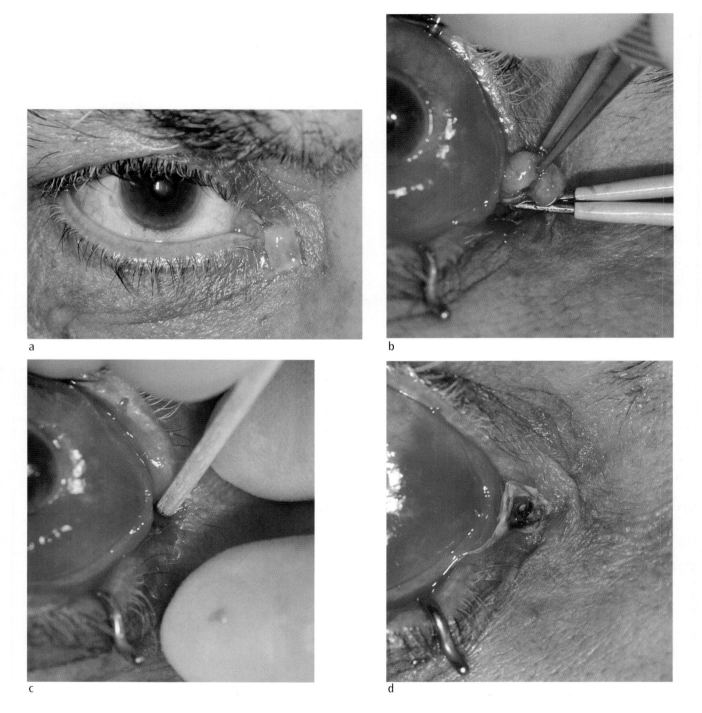

a

b

c

d

Figure 6.3

a)   Right medial canthal granuloma obscures glass tube.
b)   Local anaesthesia has been injected at medial canthus. St Martin's forceps grasp granuloma and diathermy is around neck.
c)   Silver nitrate stick application to base of papilloma. Limited application around neck of tube only.
d)   Glass tube now visible.

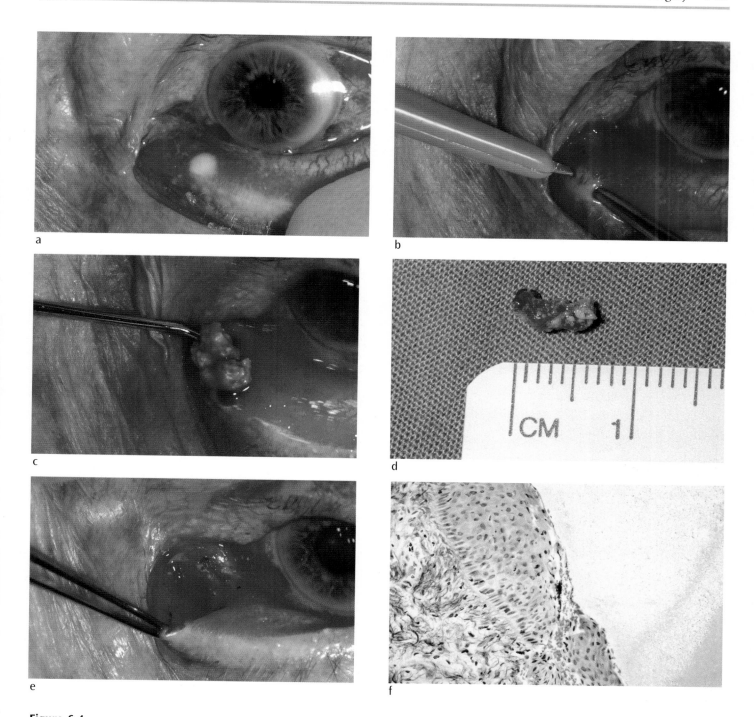

Figure 6.4

Left chronic actinomyces canaliculitis.
a)   Pouting punctum with milky discharge. Inflammation medial to punctum.
b)   Nettleship dilator inserted. Cut down medial to lateral over dilator to expose intra-canalicular concretions.
c)   Large concretion removed.
d)   Measures 7 × 3 mm.
e)   Inspect dilated mid-canaliculus, then irrigate remaining canaliculus.
f)   Histopathology of fungal canaliculitis. High power showing fungal hyphae embedded in canalicular mucosal surface. Girocott stain ×400.

Clinical features of actinomycoses canaliculitis:
- Unilateral, affects upper or lower canaliculus
- Conjunctivitis
- Discharge from pouting punctum or yellow drop at punctum (can squeeze yellow concretions out of canaliculus)
- Inflammation (redness) and swelling is medial to punctum
- Canaliculus and lacrimal system usually patent
- Widely dilated proximal or mid-canaliculus, with sulphur granules or concretions.

Management

This is by canaliculotomy under local anaesthesia (Figure 6.4).

Practice point: Topical penicillin is usually ineffective.

Post-operative management: Prescribe antibiotic steroid drops for 2 weeks. Review patient 6 weeks later, and syringe. The edges of the slit canaliculus heal well. Distal canalicular obstruction occurs rarely.

Part B: Acute canalicular trauma

Aetiology and location

Accidental injury from direct laceration (sharp) or tractional avulsion (blunt)

Age group: Young persons mainly.

Causes: Assault/fight, fall/collision, sports/stick, road traffic accident, dog bite.

Practice point: There is usually no tissue loss, except for dog bites.

Location: This occurs with eyelid injuries medial to the punctum. The lower canaliculus is affected more often than the upper canaliculus (between 3 and 5 : 1), and both the upper and lower canaliculi are involved in less than 15 per cent of canalicular injuries.

If the horizontal canaliculus is divided into thirds (lateral, mid- and medial), the mid-canalicular lacerations are more commonly caused by sharp objects and the medial lacerations from eyelid avulsion. Apparently minor medial eyelid lacerations can conceal extensive canalicular laceration, from a combined sharp and avulsion injury. The medial canthal tendon may be avulsed with the most medial canalicular injuries, together with the common canaliculus deep to it. The lacrimal sac is rarely involved. The nasolacrimal duct is usually only involved with maxillary bone injuries.

Surgical trauma

Age group: Older persons.

Causes: Surgery such as excision of a medial canthal basal cell carcinoma.

Location: Loss of a part or all of the canaliculus and punctum, and sometimes the common canaliculus. Lower and upper canaliculi are often involved. The lacrimal sac within the lacrimal fossa is usually spared.

Principles of management of accidental trauma

Suspicion

For all periocular and eyelid trauma, maintain a high suspicion of associated orbital, eye, lacrimal or brain injury. It is not the aim of this book to deal with the management of associated injuries, other than to emphasize not missing them!
- If orbital trauma is suspected, CT scan the orbits with 2–3 mm cuts, axial and direct coronal views, bone and soft tissue windows settings. MRI is useful for intra-orbital wood and other non-ferrous foreign bodies.
- If there is an eyelid laceration, assume there is a globe laceration.

- If there is a medial eyelid or medial canthal injury, assume there is lacrimal system laceration.
- If there is both eyelid and medial canthal injury, assume there is brain penetration.

Practice point: The clinical examination of orbital and head injuries should exclude CSF rhinorrhoea (cribiform plate fracture) and sub-tympanic membrane haemorrhage (petrous temporal bone fracture).

Documentation

Precise documentation of the injuries and repair, including external photography, is essential for medico-legal reasons.

Examination under anaesthetic

Immediate eyelid repair is not mandatory, but the suspicion of associated ocular injury often makes early examination under anaesthesia necessary. If there is definitely no ocular involvement, eyelid and canalicular repair should be within 3 days of the injury. The canaliculus is often easier to find 36–48 hours after the injury, once surrounding orbicularis swelling is reduced.

Eyelid injuries can be severe yet the lacrimal system preserved. For thorough examination and a good repair, exploration under general anaesthesia is required in preference to repair in the accident and emergency theatre under local anaesthesia (Figure 6.5).

Approach to trauma

1. Confirm the extent of injury and carry out primary ocular repair as indicated
2. Examine the eyelids to confirm canalicular damage and exclude tissue loss
3. Clean wound of debris; do little or no tissue debridement
4. Lower canalicular injury: repair eyelid lamellae, reconstruct canaliculus, and monocanalicular intubation
5. Upper canalicular injury: repair eyelid lamellae, reconstruct canaliculus, and monocanalicular intubation for practice

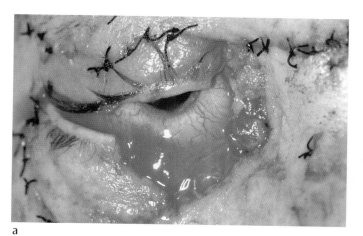

a

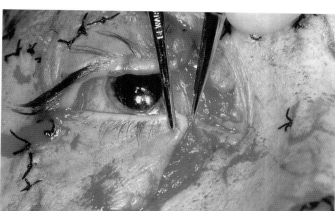

b

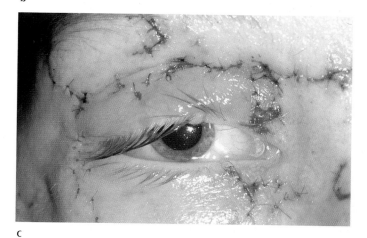

c

Figure 6.5

Trauma example 1. This young lady was in a road traffic accident in Morocco. The injuries had been partially repaired abroad, and the eyelids did not fully close.
a) Periorbital and eyelid injuries.
b) Examination under general anaesthetic revealed minimal loss of soft tissue and uninvolved canaliculi on the right.
c) The appearance 5 days after secondary repair.

6. Upper and lower canalicular injury: repair eyelid lamellae and attempt to repair at least the lower canaliculus, plus monocanalicular or bicanalicular intubation
7. Reconstruct the posterior part of the medial canthal tendon as required.

Why reconstruct monocanalicular lacerations?

This is controversial. Retrospective studies have shown that only 0–25 per cent of patients will have symptomatic epiphora when an isolated inferior canalicular laceration is *not* repaired. The upper canaliculus drains at least 30 per cent of tears when the lacrimal pump is functioning normally.

Linberg studied the effect of temporary canalicular occlusion in normal volunteers (Linberg and Moore, 1988). He inserted dissolvable hydroxypropyl cellulose punctal plugs into either the upper or lower punctum. He found that 63 per cent of subjects with experimental lower canalicular and 56 per cent with upper canalicular obstruction had symptoms of blurred vision from an increased tear film and/or sensation of a watering eye, but none had a constant watering eye. He concluded that basal tear secretion was adequately drained by one canaliculus, but that this was inadequate for reflex tears. He showed a surprisingly high rate of symptoms following upper canalicular obstruction, suggesting that these lacerations should not be ignored and that repair should be attempted.

Practice point: Since it is not possible to predict who will get symptoms and who will not, reconstruction of all canalicular lacerations is recommended.

TIP

If you decide not to reconstruct a lower monocanalicular injury (laissez-faire), you must do a good lamella eyelid repair. When the lower eyelid and punctum are in the correct anatomical position and there is a strong orbicularis, the lacrimal pump will function well and propel the tear meniscus to the medial tear lake, where it will be presented to the upper punctum for drainage. The upper punctum cannot drain the tears well if the lower eyelid is left sagging or lax.

How to repair a lacerated canaliculus

1. Location of the canaliculus
   ● Use an operating microscope or loupes to locate the cut ends of the canaliculus. The medial cut end will be circular, with rolled pale edges and visible shiny mucosa.
   ● Injection techniques (rarely needed). (a) Air injection with medial saline bath. Submerge the medial canthus in saline and inject air into the unaffected canaliculus and observe where the air bubbles emerge – it is sometimes necessary to press on lacrimal sac to close the nasolacrimal duct route. (b) Sodium hyaluronate injection into the unaffected canaliculus is an alternative to (a).
   ● Vasoconstriction of the surrounding soft tissue. Apply guttae phenylephrine 2.5–10%, adrenaline 1 in 1000, or cocaine 4–10%.

TIP

Avoid a pigtail probe as it risks damaging healthy mucosa, particularly if the barbed probe is used. Also, it is not useful if there are separate canalicular openings and hence no common canaliculus.

2. Pericanalicular repair and medial canthal tendon repair:
   ● Support the canalicular repair and restore the eyelid position by suturing the cut orbicularis with 6.0 Vicryl and the tough posterior MCT limb with 6.0 Vicryl or 5.0 non-absorbable suture. Place the sutures on bulldog clips and delay tying them until after the canalicular sutures have been positioned.
3. Canalicular repair:
   ● Use fine 8.0 absorbable sutures inserted into each end of the torn canaliculus with the aid of a microscope or loupes.
4. Intubation (probing or dilating the canaliculus, prior to silicone tube insertion facilitates the procedure):
   ● Use a soft, inert, pliable, silicone stent.
   ● If it is a monocanalicular laceration, use monocanalicular self-retaining intubation. This has no risks to the unaffected canaliculus and does not intubate the nasolacrimal duct, but its trimmed end lies in the lacrimal sac.
   ● If it is a bicanalicular laceration, use bicanalicular intubation – prepare the nose to

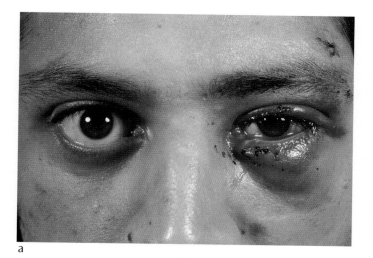

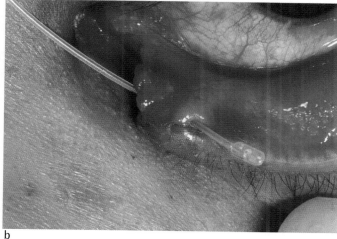

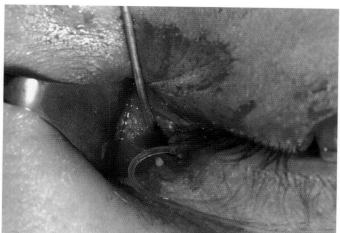

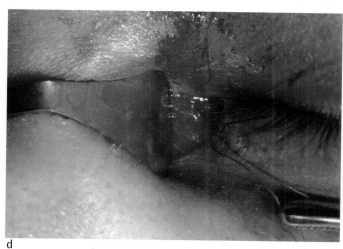

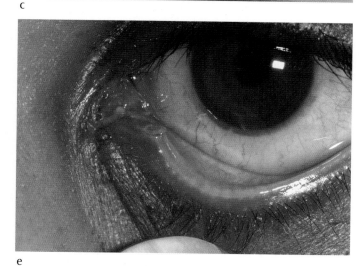

Figure 6.6

Trauma example 2. Young man with left upper and lower eyelid lacerations following a fight. The lower canalicular laceration was reconstructed and the patient did not have subsequent epiphora.

a) Confirm an avulsion injury with a mid-canalicular to medial canalicular laceration.

b) Dilate the punctum and insert a Mini-monaka self-retaining silicone tube through it, which localizes the lateral cut end.

c) Retract the medial soft tissue with Fison's retractor and probe the medial end of cut canaliculus. Dilate the medial end and open it slightly with a blade if this helps.

d) Pass two absorbable sutures through the substantia propria of each cut canalicular end. Pre-place one or two 6.0 absorbable sutures in the deep orbicularis and medial canthal tendon to the posterior lacrimal crest. Trim the end of the Mini-monaka and place its end in the lacrimal sac. Now tighten and secure the surrounding sutures. Use 6.0 absorbable sutures to the anterior orbicularis and 6.0 black silk or Novafil to the skin.

e) Appearance of left medial canthus and lower eyelid 4 weeks later. There is minimal mucus production and the Mini-monaka is self-retaining.

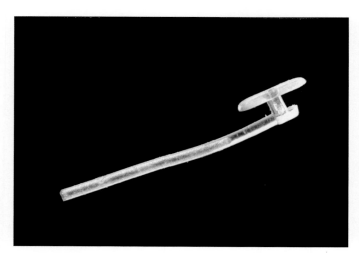

Figure 6.7

The tube was left in for 3 months and then removed by simply pulling it out. Note that it was just long enough to reach into the sac.

receive the tubes from the nasolacrimal duct into the inferior meatus under direct endoscopic view.
5. Post-operative pressure dressing:
    ● Apply a compression dressing for 24–48 hours after surgery to reduce swelling, taped to reduce wound tension.
6. Removal of the tube:
    ● Remove the silicone tube after 1–3 months.

See Figures 6.6–6.9.

Medial versus lateral canalicular injuries

Medial canalicular avulsions are more difficult to repair than lateral canalicular lacerations.

With medial canalicular lacerations, repair the thin posterior sheet of medial canthal tendon by passing a 6.0 absorbable or 5.0 permanent Ethibond suture towards the posterior lacrimal crest, deep to the sac. This is the MCT posterior fixation suture (Figure 6.10). It may be necessary to open the conjunctiva between the caruncle and plica semilunaris to find the correct plane. Do not shorten the lid margin length by overdoing the repair.

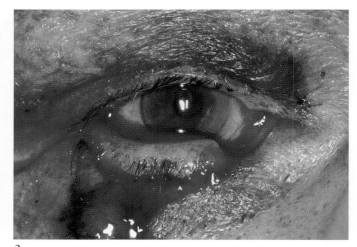

a

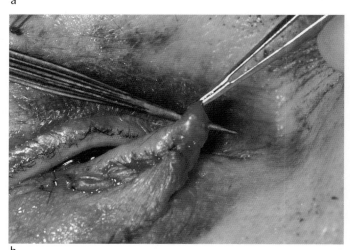

b

Figure 6.8

Trauma example 3. This elderly man fell over a curb and lacerated his lower eyelid. He had a lateral canalicular laceration, which was reconstructed and intubated. There was no epiphora after removal of the tube, and syringing was patent with no noticeable narrowing.
a) Inspect eyelid and medial canthus to confirm extent of injury.
b) Dilate the lower punctum and identify the lateral cut end of the lower canaliculus.
c) Retract the medial soft tissue and identify the pale appearance of the medial cut end of the lower canaliculus.
d) Pass a trimmed Mini-monaka tube through the lateral part of the canaliculus.
e) Three 8.0 absorbable Vicryl sutures are pre-placed into the substantia propria of the medial canalicular end, then the lateral canalicular end.
f) Repair the eyelid posterior lamella with 6.0 absorbable Vicryl and pass the tube into the sac. Tighten all sutures and secure.
g) Close the anterior orbicularis with 6.0 Vicryl and skin with 6.0 non-absorbable Novafil.
h) Appearance at end of repair.

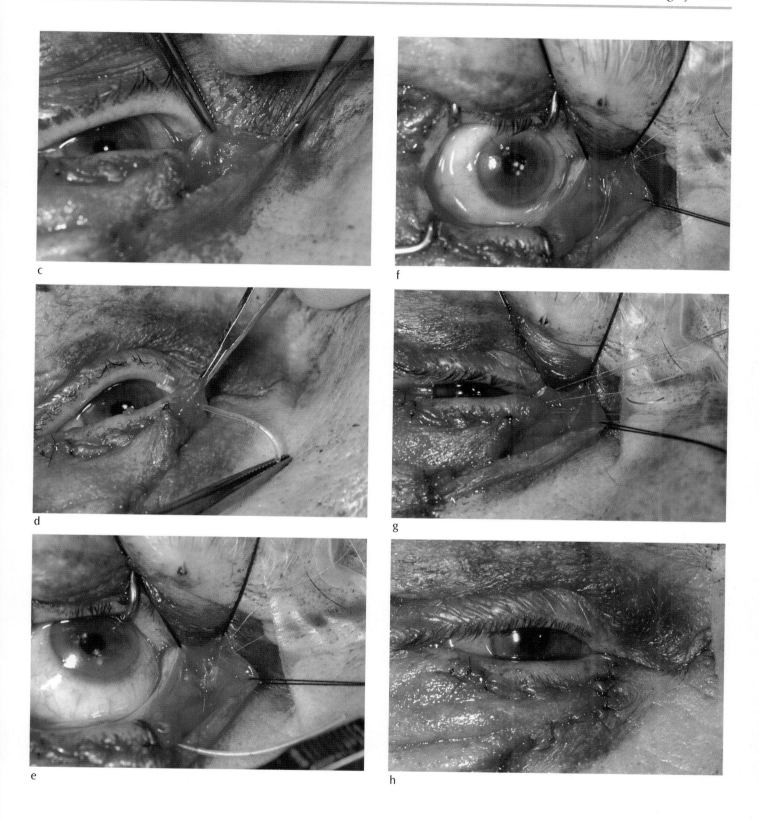

c

d

e

f

g

h

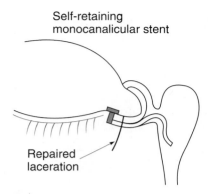

Figure 6.9

Diagram showing position of monocanalicular stent in lower canalicular reconstruction.

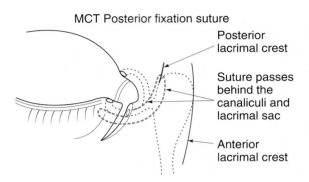

Figure 6.10

Diagram showing position of posterior fixation suture from medial end of tarsal plate to posterior lacrimal crest.

If the laceration is very medial or involves the common canaliculus, it is difficult to identify the medial cut end. It may be necessary to do a DCR with retrograde intubation. This is the exception where a pigtail probe can be tried gently before DCR.

Lateral canalicular lacerations are easier to repair as the medial end can be identified by its pale colour, and the medial canthal tendon does not need posterior fixation (as in Figure 6.8).

Canalicular marsupialization

This is a canaliculostomy or exteriorization of the medial cut end of the lacerated canaliculus into the conjunctival sac. The eyelid lamella and posterior limb of the MCT are repaired as above. If possible, stent as for canalicular repair. This technique is particularly useful for medial canthal repair after tumour excision. It can also be used after accidental trauma (Figures 6.11, 6.12).

Combined upper and lower canalicular injuries

These are more difficult to manage, and have a high risk of permanent epiphora. Aim for reconstruction with bicanalicular nasolacrimal duct intubation. Alternatively, aim for a good lower canalicular reconstruction with monocanalicular intubation and careful upper medial eyelid repair.

Other lacrimal system injuries

Lacrimal sac: Acute injuries are rare; either explore immediately and do DCR, or wait and do late repair. There may be associated telecanthus requiring late transnasal wire.

Nasolacrimal duct: Associated bony injury, therefore do late DCR after maxillo-facial surgery.

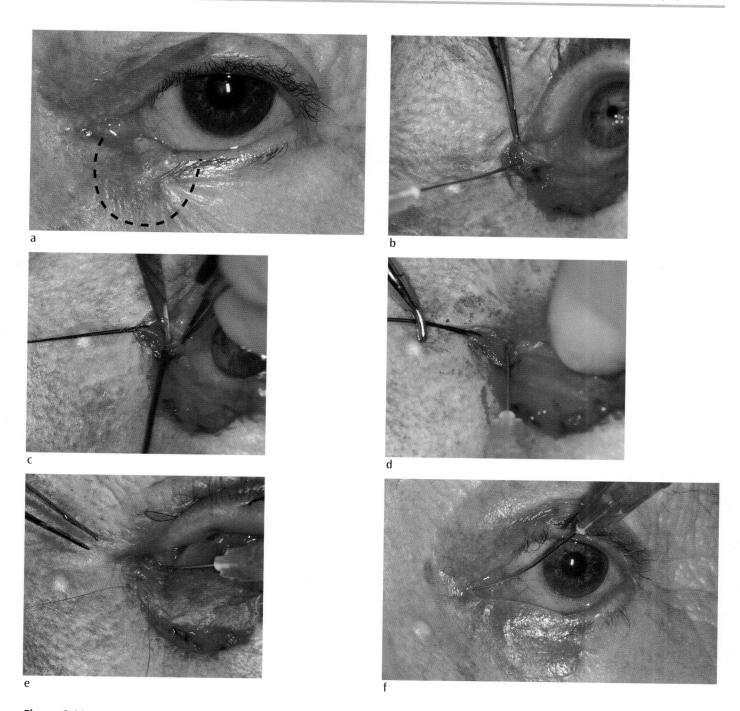

Figure 6.11

Canalicular marsupialization.

a)   Recurrent lower medial eyelid basal cell carcinoma. Approximate area for excision marked.

b)   Post-Mohs' micrographic surgery, the medial cut end of the lower canaliculus is identified and irrigated.

c)   Anterior traction suture helps exposure. The medial cut end is probed, then a no. 11 blade is used to cut down onto the posterior aspect of the canaliculus.

d)   The widened canaliculus is irrigated.

e)   Reconstruction of defect by a Hughes tarso-conjunctival flap with free skin graft. The posterior edge of the lateral end of the widened canaliculus is sutured open to the edge of the conjunctival flap and skin edge using 8.0 absorbable suture.

f)   Three months after repair and opening of the flap, the patient has no epiphora and the marsupialized lower canaliculus is easily irrigating.

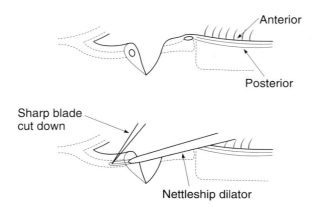

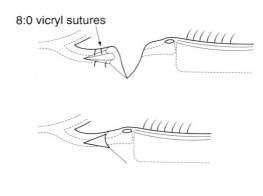

Figure 6.12

Diagram showing canalicular marsupialization into conjunctival fornix.

Part C: Longstanding canalicular obstruction

General guidelines:

- If there is more than 8 mm of functioning canaliculus measured from the punctum, a canaliculo-DCR is done.
- If there is less than 8 mm of functioning canaliculus measured from the punctum, a conjunctivo-DCR with bypass tube is done.

In practice there are many different patterns of canalicular obstruction, and the extent is not always initially known from simple probing or dacryocystography and can only be gauged by exploration with retrograde probing via the common canalicular opening. For instance, if there is 5 mm of functioning canaliculus measured from the punctum with a focal mid-canalicular obstruction and healthy distal canaliculus, do a DCR and attempt retrograde intubation. If there is a 5 mm proximal lower canalicular *obstruction* and a patent distal canaliculus, do a DCR with retrograde intubation and exteriorization of the remaining patent medial canaliculus.

Even though the nasolacrimal duct is often completely normal in the presence of canalicular disease, a DCR is invariably done (unless doing endocanalicular surgery) in order to provide access to the lacrimal sac lumen and common canalicular opening and reduce outflow resistance. Alternatively, see Chapter 8, p. 196, Adult nasolacrimal duct intubation.

Patterns of canalicular obstruction (Figure 6.13)

1. Proximal (lateral) common canaliculus (CC) fibrosis
2. Distal (medial) common canaliculus (CC) membranous obstruction from chronic sac disease
3. Focal distal (medial) and mid-canalicular fibrosis
4. Mid- and/or distal (medial) canalicular
   - Generalized
   - Focal
5. Proximal (lateral) canalicular.

Canalicular surgery

There is a range of types of surgery, all with silicone intubation:

1. (a) Canaliculo- and common canaliculo-DCR, or

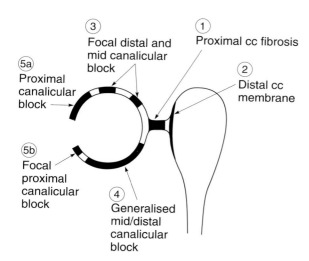

Figure 6.13

Diagram showing types of canalicular obstruction.

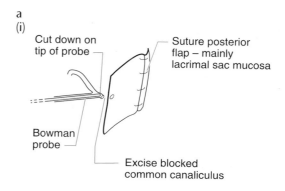

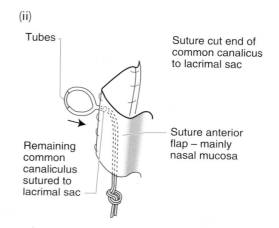

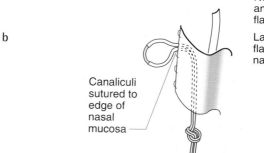

Figure 6.14

Diagrams showing principles of a) i) and ii) common canaliculo-DCR and b) canalicular rhinostomy.

(b) canaliculo- and common canaliculo-rhinostomy (no sac present)
2. Common internal punctoplasty/membranectomy
3. DCR with retrograde canaliculostomy
4. Endolacrimal canaliculotomy.

Canaliculo- and common canaliculo-DCR; canaliculo- and common canaliculo-rhinostomy

An anastomosis is made between the medial ends of the canaliculi or the common canaliculus and the nasal mucosa; therefore 'canaliculo-DCR or common canaliculo-DCR' are the correct terms (Figure 6.14a). The lacrimal sac mucosa is used to make the posterior flap. If no lacrimal sac mucosa is present, the correct terms are 'canaliculo-rhinostomy or common canaliculo-rhinostomy' (Figure 6.14b), and the nasal mucosa is used to make a very large anterior flap. Temporary silicone intubation is placed for up to 3–4 months. The success rate for a common canaliculo-DCR is approximately 80 per cent, and for a canaliculo-DCR is approximately 60 per cent. If the lacrimal sac is merely fibrosed rather than lost from tumour, it may be possible to salvage adequate mucosa to create a flap when the rhinostomy is enlarged anteriorly; otherwise canaliculo- or common canaliculo-rhinostomy is required. These have success rates in the range of 40 per cent.

Indications

1. Upper and lower distal (medial) canalicular obstruction (8 mm remaining)
2. Proximal (lateral) common canalicular fibrosis
3. Small scarred sac or no lacrimal sac, e.g. after dacryocystectomy or medial canthal tumour excision.

Principles of surgery

Identify the canaliculi lateral to the tear sac and resect the obstruction. Use a loupe or an operating microscope. An extra large rhinostomy is made for mobilization of a large nasal mucosal flap.

Technique

The precise steps depend on individual surgical findings, but guidelines are as follows:

- Use a standard external approach skin incision (lateral side of nose or tear trough) with division of the anterior limb of the medial canthal tendon close to the maxilla bone.
- Place the medial canthal tendon on a lateral traction suture.
- Insert Bowman probes or an angled Werb probe into the upper and lower canaliculi, keeping them horizontal (in the plane of the iris). Hold the medial canthal tendon on its traction suture and reflect it laterally. Dissect gently under the tendon and cut down onto the tips of the probes at the most medial point they reach, lateral to the sac. Remove overlying scar tissue.
- If lacrimal sac is present, open it very anterior (sac mucosa will form the posterior flap).
- Use retrograde probing to confirm obstruction or patency of the common canaliculus.
- Resect fibrosed canaliculus/common canaliculus.
- Intubate both canaliculi and any remaining common canaliculus.
- Re-attach the cut ends of the canaliculi or remaining common canaliculus to the lacrimal sac with 8.0 Vicryl, using loupes/microscope.
- Make an extra large rhinostomy (20 mm in diameter) and expose healthy nasal mucosa (large anterior flap). If a previous DCR has been done, first locate the edges of the old rhinostomy and then enlarge it anterior – you will always be able to find healthy nasal mucosa! Then remove the plug of scar tissue in the old rhinostomy.
- Suture the posterior flap (mainly lacrimal sac).
- Suture the anterior flap (mainly nasal mucosa). If there is no lacrimal sac, the nasal mucosa alone makes the anterior flap, sutured to anterior lamella tissue, and the posterior flap is omitted.
- Perform standard MCT and skin flap closure.

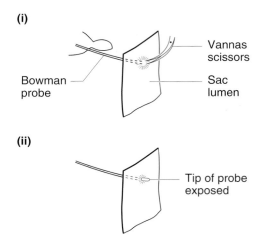

Figure 6.15

Diagram showing internal membranectomy at DCR.

Common canalicular internal punctoplasty or membranectomy

A thin membrane at the medial end of the common canaliculus is approached from inside the sac and excised (Figure 6.15). The success rate is approximately 90 per cent.

Indications

Distal (medial) membranous common canalicular obstruction.

Technique

Do a standard DCR. When the sac is open, use the Bowman probe to tent up the membrane obstructing the common opening at the medial end of the common canaliculus and incise. Cut down onto the probe with a sharp blade, laser or fine Vannas scissors. Excise excess membrane. Intubate with temporary silicone tubes for 6–12 weeks, depending on the severity.

DCR with retrograde canaliculostomy and intubation

This is retrograde exploration of the canaliculi with a false passage (false punctum) made for intubation

(Figure 6.16). The aim of this operation is to try and avoid a Lester Jones bypass tube. Approximately 70 per cent of patients have improved symptoms, but only 20 per cent of these are completely asymptomatic.

> Practice point: Retrograde intubation is not easy to do.

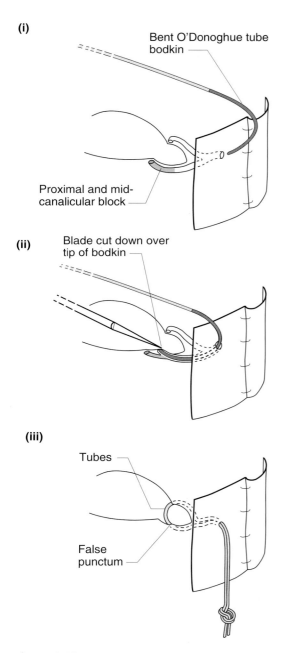

(i)

Bent O'Donoghue tube bodkin

Proximal and mid-canalicular block

(ii)

Blade cut down over tip of bodkin

(iii)

Tubes

False punctum

Figure 6.16

Diagram showing DCR with retrograde intubation.

Indications

Focal mid and proximal canalicular obstruction.

Principles of surgery

Open the lacrimal sac for access to the common canalicular opening for retrograde intubation via a standard external approach DCR.

Technique

Do a standard external approach DCR skin incision with a large rhinostomy (20 mm in diameter), open the lacrimal sac and prepare the nasal flaps in the standard way. Suture the posterior mucosal flaps to reduce bleeding.

- Use an operating microscope, rigid nasal endoscope or loupes to identify the common canalicular opening. If only one canaliculus is obstructed, identify the opening by antegrade probing of the normal canaliculus.
- Bend the metal bodkin attached to the silicone tubes for retrograde insertion into the common canalicular opening, and then towards the obstructed canaliculus. Alternatively, bend a Bowman probe (size 0) and locate and probe the common opening before antrograde intubation.
- Palpate the position of the tip along the canaliculus and use a Barde Parker no.11 blade or other sharp blade to cut down onto the probe on the supero-posterior surface. This creates a pseudo-punctum (canaliculotomy).
- Once the false punctum has been fashioned, perform either retrograde or simple antrograde intubation via the pseudo-punctum with O'Donoghue tubes.
- Complete the standard DCR.
- Remove the tubes after 2–3 months.

Endolacrimal canaliculotomy with intubation

Endocanalicular surgery is a rapidly evolving area in which stenoses within the canaliculi are detected and lasered using a holmium, erbium or KTP laser (Figure 6.17).

Endocanalicular surgery

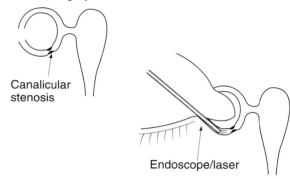

Figure 6.17

Diagram of endolacrimal canaliculoplasty.

Indications

Focal intra-canalicular obstruction with or without nasolacrimal obstruction.

Technique

● Use guttae cocaine to vasoconstrict the canalicular mucosa.
● Probe and irrigate each canaliculus to locate the stenosis.
● Insert the endocanalicular probe (diameter 0.8 or 0.9 mm) to visualize the abnormality.
● Position the laser probe (erbium, holmium or KTP laser) and advance gently towards the stenosis. Laser the stenosis. This is not always under direct vision, and the best laser and settings to use are yet to be established.
● Probe and irrigate the canaliculus to confirm treated stenosis, wash out any blood or debris and confirm patent nasolacrimal duct.
● Re-inspect canaliculi with endoprobe.
● If the nasolacrimal duct is not patent, perform endocanalicular or endonasal laser DCR.
● Insert bicanalicular intubation with inferior meatus retrieval under direct endoscopic endonasal view if done without associated DCR, or pass through the rhinostomy if DCR is done.
● Leave the tubes in for 8–16 weeks, depending on the lesion treated.

TIP

Try one of the above procedures before committing the patient to a conjunctivo-DCR with bypass tube, unless there is obviously severe proximal and mid-canalicular obstruction with less than 8 mm of functioning canaliculus. If canalicular surgery fails, place a Jones tube.

Canalicular bypass surgery

Conjunctivodacryocystorhinostomy (CDCR) with the insertion of a Lester Jones pyrex glass bypass tube is a procedure which creates a lacrimal drainage route from the conjunctiva into the nasal space, bypassing the canaliculi and sac. The proximal end of the Jones tube lies at the medial canthus, and the distal end at the anterior end of the middle meatus. It passes through soft tissue and a DCR rhinostomy.

Indications for Jones bypass tube

1. Less than 8 mm of patent canaliculus from the punctum (e.g. extensive proximal canalicular obstruction, congenital or acquired agenesis)
2. Failed canaliculo-DCR or other canalicular surgery
3. Functional epiphora, e.g. facial palsy.

Aetiology of extensive canalicular obstruction treated by Jones bypass tubes:
• Medial canthal and lacrimal system trauma/radiotherapy (Figure 6.18)
• Herpes simplex canaliculitis
• Congenital punctal and canalicular agenesis
• Failed canaliculo-DCR or other canalicular surgery
• Other, rarer causes including:
  • Chlamydial infection
  • Stevens–Johnson syndrome
  • Systemic high dose 5-fluorouracil
  • Trachoma
  • Herpes zoster
  • Following medial canthal tumour excision with loss of lacrimal system
  • Medial canthal burns or radiotherapy
  • Functional epiphora in facial palsy, after other surgery
  • Centurion syndrome
  • Idiopathic.

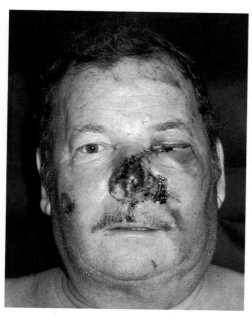

Figure 6.18

Severe left canalicular and sac trauma associated with facial and medial canthal injuries. This patient required a transnasal wiring and left eye enucleation. An exploratory DCR with retrograde intubation failed. He had a successful secondary endoscopic endonasal placement of a Lester–Jones tube.

Jones bypass tube placement

Jones bypass tube placement used to be done with external DCR, but is now more often done as a primary or secondary endonasal endoscopic assisted procedure (Table 6.1).

1. Primary placement of Jones tube
    ● with external DCR
    ● with endoscopic endonasal surgical or laser DCR.

2. Secondary closed placement of Jones tube with endonasal monitoring.
3. Replacement Jones tube.

Caruncle or eyelid tube placement?

Options:
1. Transcanalicular (lower eyelid, medial to the punctum)
2. Pre-canalicular
    ● Anterior medial canthal angle (anterior caruncle)
    ● Inferior-anterior caruncle.

If there is a wide lower punctum and functioning proximal canaliculus, eyelid placement functions well. Open the first 5 mm and put the tube in the posterior lamella of the eyelid. The cosmetic appearance is excellent, but the disadvantage is that a longer tube is required and there is poor retention in the soft tissue, with a greater tendency for the tube to fall out.

Medial canthal or caruncle placement has greater stability, uses a shorter tube and has a lower tube loss rate, but there is a risk of the tube burying in. Only remove part of the caruncle if it is really necessary.

Accurate placement

Pre-operative evaluation of the nasal space
This assists in the early identification of potential problems and correct planning of surgery. Unidentified endonasal anatomical factors could lead to drainage failure from occlusion of the distal end of the tube. For instance, a significantly deviated septum with a narrow

Table 6.1 Jones bypass surgery

	Indication	Method	Alternative method
Primary placement of Jones tube	Extensive canalicular obstruction	Endoscopic endonasal laser or surgical DCR and closed Jones tube placement	External DCR and open Jones tube placement
Secondary placement of Jones tube	After failed canalicular surgery with DCR	Surgical endonasal endoscopic assisted closed placement	
Replacement	If tube is lost or buried in	Remove tube and replace with endonasal endoscopic assisted closed technique	

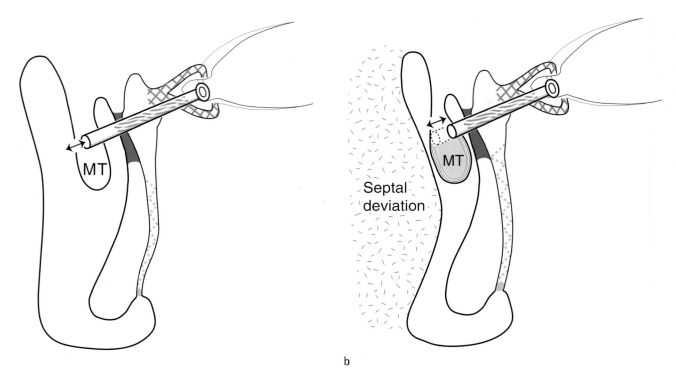

a   b

Figure 6.19

a)   Diagram showing good position of Jones tube within a wide nasal space. There is ample endonasal space for tube movement (rocking) during blinking.

b)   The nasal space is narrow secondary to septal deviation and a large concha bullosa, but there is still adequate endonasal space for tube movement. There may be intermittent tube-septum touch but tube-septal impaction is unlikely.

nasal space provides poor access to the middle turbinate and meatus, and little space for the distal end of the tube. A planned submucosal resection of a prominent septum by a rhinological colleague, before or at the time of Jones tube placement, may be indicated. Normal anatomical variations such as a large concha bullosa or pathological findings such as traumatic synaechiae and polyps should be identified, as they may require division or limited turbinectomy.

TIP

If the nasal space is very narrow, ask a rhinology colleague to do a submucosal resection of the septum to create room to examine the distal end of the tube per and post-operatively.

Direction of tube insertion

The tube should be directed from the lower eyelid or anterior caruncle, 30–45° infero-medially into the nose.

If the tube is directed too steeply downwards, the direction and its weight will make it more prone to burying in. The length of the tube must be accurately assessed, since too short a tube will bury in proximally and too long a tube may extrude proximally or abut distally on the septum, and fail. Nasal endoscopic monitoring of the distal end is essential before, during and after tube placement. The medial end of the tube should lie in the lacrimal lake and the distal end approximately 2–3 mm from the septal mucosa (Figure 6.19).

Techniques for Jones tube placement

In primary placement a standard external DCR with a large rhinostomy is performed, where the nasal space can be visualized both directly and endoscopically. Primary laser endonasal endoscopic DCR enables rapid

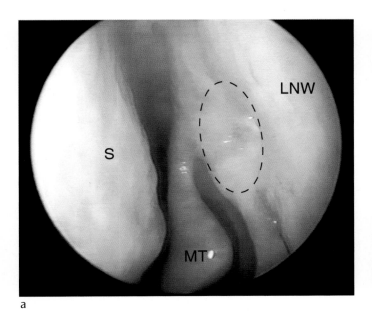
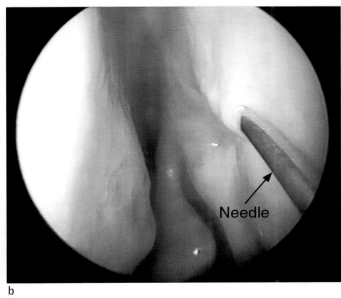

a   b

Figure 6.20

Secondary Jones tube placement.
a)   The previous DCR site is outlined – in this area there is no intervening bone, only soft tissue.
b)   Local anaesthesia injected into lateral nasal wall.

tube placement and provides a tight ostium around the tube, which may provide greater stability. In those cases where an initial canaliculo-DCR or related type of operation has failed and there is already a bony rhinostomy, secondary placement is easy.

Secondary (surgical) Jones tube placement

This is done under local or general anaesthesia, with standard nasal mucosal preparation as for other endonasal lacrimal surgery (Figure 6.20).

- Place K-wire. A 1.1 mm diameter Kirshner-wire (K-wire) is placed via the posterior eyelid medial to the punctum or the anterior/inferior caruncle, directed through the rhinostomy. In caruncle placement, some surgeons recommend partial caruncle excision prior to placement. When placing the K-wire, keep it in the plane of the iris, directed 30–45° infero-medially, and view it emerging into the nose (Figure 6.21).

TIP

The K-wire is sharp at both ends, so be very careful with your fingers and those of your assistant.

- Trephine out soft tissue. Use a fine (1.5 or 2.0 mm) trephine to remove a core of soft tissue around the K-wire. Do this twice to make a slightly larger tract. Sometimes the K-wire is removed with the trephine and then replaced for the second trephining to make the tract wider. View endonasally with the Hopkins endoscope to confirm correct positioning. Use the trephine depth to measure the length of tube required. Keep the K-wire in for tube placement (Figure 6.22).
- Pass the Jones tube over the K-wire. After selecting the correct length tube (usually 14–18 mm long and flange 3–4 mm diameter), thread the tube over the wire and push it down the soft tissue tract into the nose, still under direct endoscopic view. Remove the K-wire, holding the Jones tube in place. Observe tears dripping out of the tube, or irrigate to demonstrate this (Figures 6.23, 6.24).

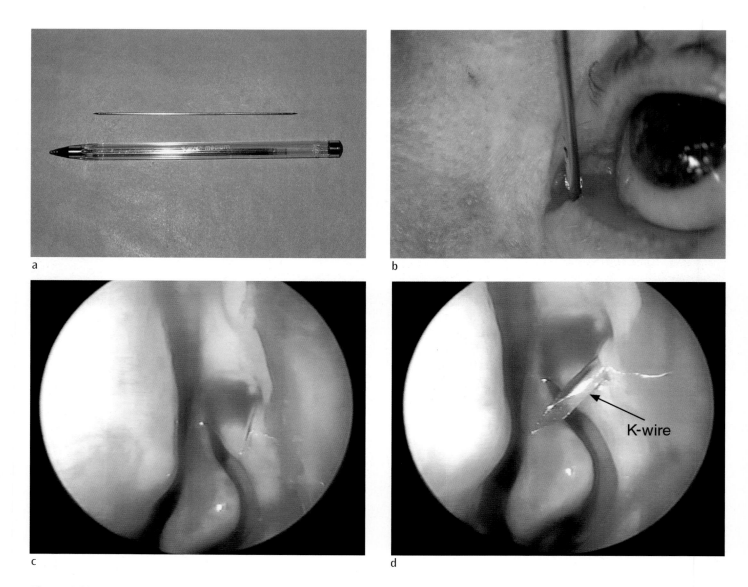

Figure 6.21

a)   K-wire. Note size of wire compared to biro.
b)   K-wire is passed down through the lower eyelid posterior lamella into the nose, keeping it in the plane of the iris, taking care not to direct posteriorly. This patient has an artificial eye.
c)   Tip of K-wire visible in sub-mucosa.
d)   K-wire emerging into nose through old DCR site. Correct positioning.

● Secure the tube with a Prolene suture around its neck to the eyelid. This suture is usually removed after 3 weeks. There are Lester-Jones tubes with a hole at the neck, which make suturing easier.

TIP

The tubes are hand-blown glass, and therefore some variation in diameter exists. Always keep a stock of several different length tubes and more than one of each, as sometimes the chosen tube will not pass down over the wire.

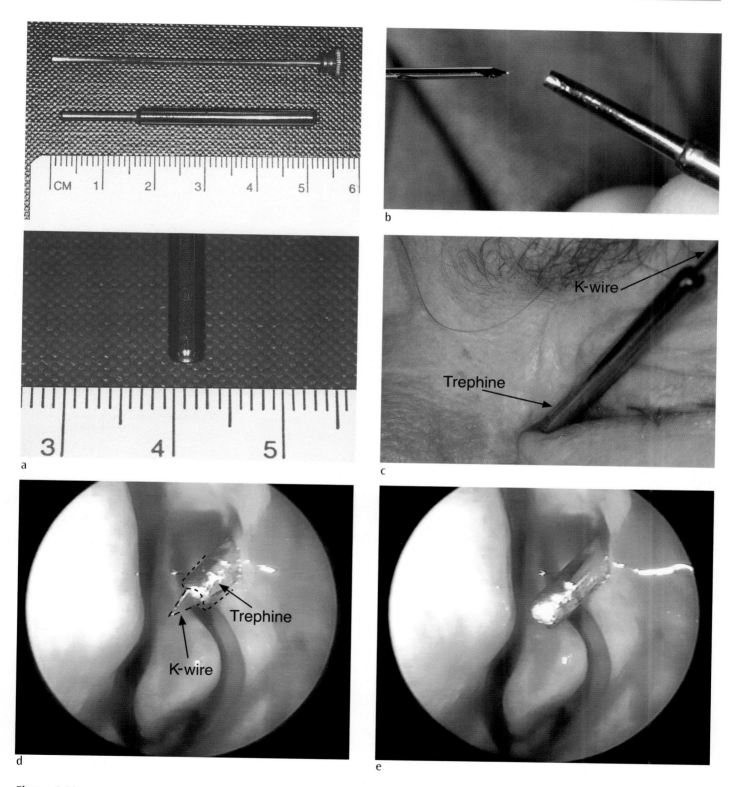

Figure 6.22

a)   5 cm long trephine and stent, and sharp tip of trephine.
b)   With the K-wire *in situ*, the trephine is threaded over it.
c)   The trephine is advanced through the soft tissue to the nose and a core of tissue removed. This is repeated.
d)   Both the K-wire and the trephine can be seen in the nose.
e)   Just the trephine is visible endonasally, as it advances past the tip of the K-wire.

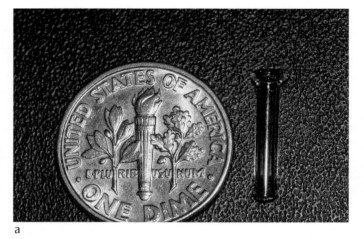

a

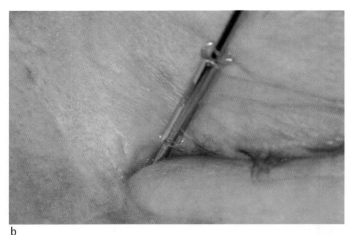

b

c

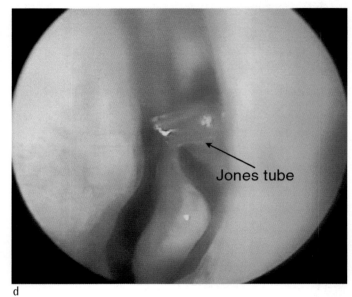

d

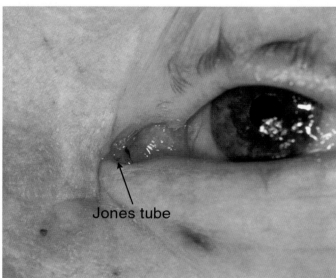

e

Figure 6.23

a) A typical glass Jones bypass tube.
b) The Jones tube is passed down over the K-wire.
c) The K-wire is removed once the tube is in place.
d) The endonasal position of the distal end of the tube is checked.
e) A tear drop is seen dripping through it, confirming function.

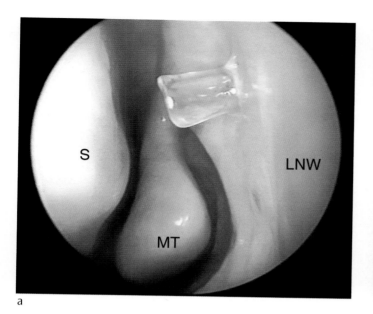
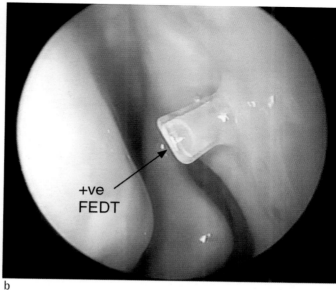

a

b

Figure 6.24

One week after secondary Jones tube placement, showing normal functional endoscopic dye test.
a)   Good tube position.
b)   Fluorescein has filled lumen and splashed inside nose.

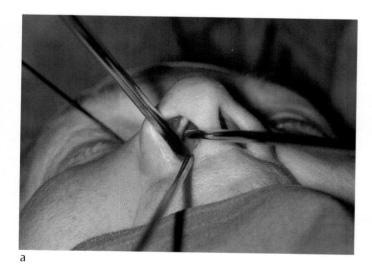
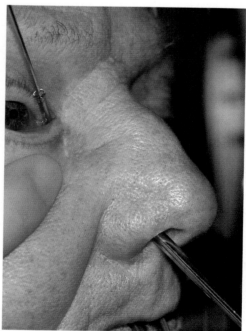

a

b

Figure 6.25

Primary holmium laser-assisted Jones tube placement.
a)   The K-wire is pushed through to the correct position on
       the lateral nasal wall, and the three instruments are in
       the nose: Hopkins endoscope, laser tip and smoke sucker.
       View of eye and nose from below.
b)   The Jones tube is passed down over the K-wire into the
       nose, with endoscopic monitoring.

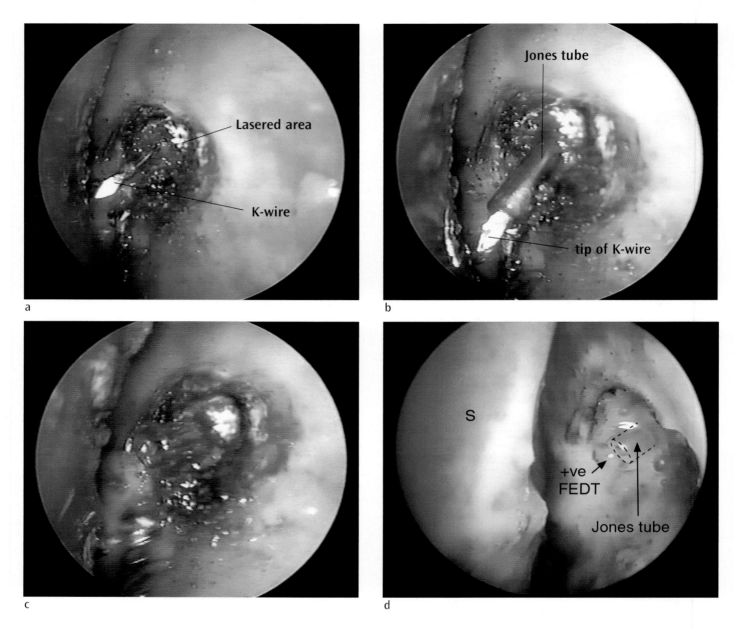

Figure 6.26 Left primary laser-assisted Jones tube placement.

a) Nasal mucosa and bone surrounding K-wire is ablated by holmium laser (10 W). Marked tissue char is noted. Alternatively, the KTP laser may be used.
b) The Jones tube is passed down over the K-wire.
c) The K-wire is removed, leaving the tube in place.
d) Appearance 1 week after surgery with positive functional endoscopic dye test.

TIP

There is no need to use laser for secondary Jones tube placement.

Primary laser-assisted Jones tube placement

The laser is used to create a channel between the nose and the anterior caruncle (Figures 6.25–6.27).

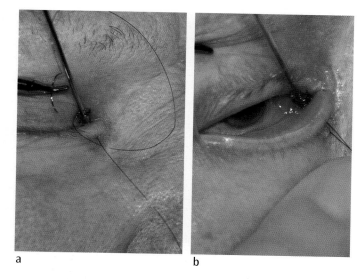

a   b

Figure 6.27

A suture is placed around the Jones tube collar to stabilize it.
a) The 6.0 Prolene suture is passed through the lower eyelid from the skin to the conjunctival surface, then wrapped around the tube collar, keeping the K-wire *in situ*.
b) The suture is brought out to the skin surface and knotted. The K-wire can then be removed.

- Push either a large needle or the K-wire through from the caruncle into the nose at the level of the middle meatus just posterior to the lacrimal ridge. The wire has to pass through thin lacrimal bone or else the lasering will be 'blind' to reach the K-wire tip through the thicker maxilla bone in the anterior part of the lacrimal sac.
- Laser ablate the mucosa and bone around the tip to create a small space for the tube.

- Use the trephine to remove a core of soft tissue around the K-wire.
- Pass the tube down over the K-wire, as above. It is sometimes necessary to push the tube down quite firmly, even using a Moorfield's forceps to push on the flange. If instruments are used, be careful not to crack the glass tube.
- Secure the tube with a temporary 6.0 Prolene suture around its collar to the lower eyelid, as above.

TIP

A small rhinostomy will hold the glass tube well.

Post-operative management of Jones tubes

Immediately after surgery

Apply steroid-antibiotic drops qds for 1–3 weeks. The patient should not blow the nose for 4 days, but should then be encouraged to blow and sniff to check tube functioning, whilst holding a finger over the medial canthus to prevent loss/extrusion of tube.

One week after surgery

Examine the tube position and function. Note the position of the proximal end on adduction and abduction, using the slit lamp. Observe fluctuations of tear movement and even air bubbles down the tube lumen, and do a functional endoscopic dye test and observe the passive drip of fluorescein from the tube, viewed endonasally with the Hopkins endoscope (Figures 6.28, 6.29).

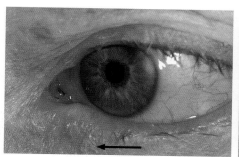
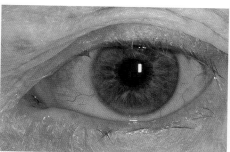
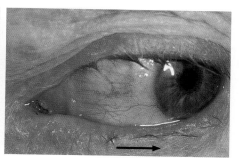

Figure 6.28

Proximal end of tube. Normal tube position in anterior inferior caruncle. There is no tube–eye touch on adduction, or displacement on abduction. This tube functions well.

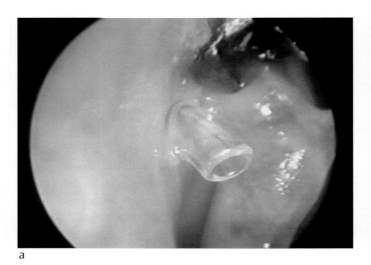
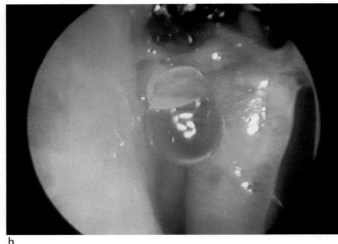

a   b

Figure 6.29

Right functioning Jones tube. Note the normal rocking movement of the distal end of the tube.
a)   Tube faces downwards and is long.
b)   Tube is horizontal and shorter. This also shows a fluorescein drop, indicating a positive functional endoscopic dye test.

Examining the tube

Examine the tube regularly, at 2–3-month intervals for up to 6 months, then at increasingly longer intervals. Inspect the position of the collar, probe and syringe the tube, and inspect the distal end endonasally, performing the functional endoscopic dye test.

The aftercare of Jones tube patients requires a good ophthalmologist–patient relationship.

Sniff test

Teach the patient how to do the sniff test. The patient holds the nose and sniffs in and out, noticing how air passes up and down the tube. The patient should be encouraged to do this daily and recognize the sound and feel of a functioning tube; if the sniff test is negative, the patient should visit the clinic urgently for tube inspection and cleaning or replacement if indicated. Similarly, if the tube falls out, the patient should return urgently (preferably with the tube!) for replacement.

Post-operative problems

The majority of patients (75–90 per cent) will be satisfied with their tube, but 50 per cent will lose or require it replacing within 5 years.

Complications of Jones bypass tubes:
1.   Tube proximal end
     • Buries in/conjunctival overgrowth
     • Displaces laterally, causing ocular irritation/erosion
     • Wrong angle causes intermittent function – e.g. only on abduction
     • Granuloma
     • Spontaneous or iatrogenic loss.
2.   Distal end
     • Nasal mucosal overgrowth obstructs drainage
     • Granuloma obstructs drainage
     • End impacts on middle turbinate or septum, giving partial or total loss of function
     • Calcium and mucous debris obstructs the lumen.

Granulation tissue at proximal end: Treat with silver nitrate stick application endonasally.

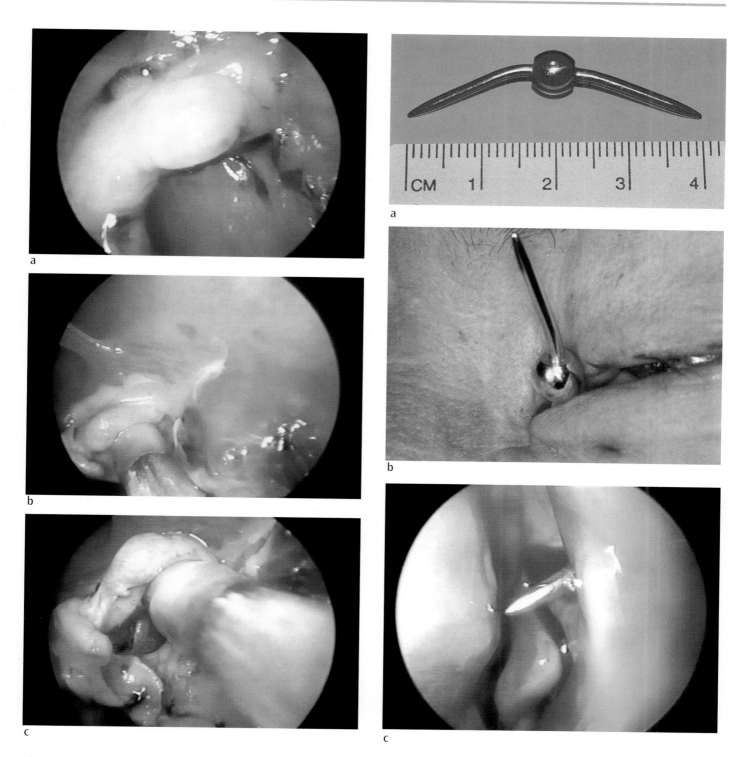

Figure 6.30

Nasal mucosal overgrowth.
a)   Left endonasal view of nasal mucosal overgrowth concealing distal end of Jones tube. Non-functioning tube.
b)   Silver nitrate stick application.
c)   The tube is becoming visible, containing fluorescein.

Figure 6.31

Replacement Jones tube.
a)   4 cm gold horn.
b)   Gold horn opens existing tract or creates new tract.
c)   Correct position of gold horn on lateral nasal wall prior to introducing tube.

Nasal mucosal overgrowth at distal end: Treat with silver nitrate stick application endonasally (Figure 6.30).

Tube impacting on septum: Replace with shorter tube and ensure that it is passed through firm tissue for stability (e.g. anterior caruncle at medial canthal angle), where the proximal end cannot bury into soft tissue. Check the angle into the nose – if it is too vertical, it can predispose to burying in and subsequent septum impaction.

Tube loss/replacement: The original tube or a new tube can be replaced easily under local anaesthesia. The nose is prepared with decongestant and local anaesthesia. The medial canthus is infiltrated with local anaesthetic, and topical anaesthetic is used on the ocular surface.

- The gold horn is used to feel for the old tract or create a new tract. Alternatively, the K-wire and trephine are used as for secondary tube placement.
- The Jones tube is pushed down the tract and its neck secured using a temporary 6.0 Prolene suture (Figure 6.31).

TIP

The gold horn is sometimes used for widening a tract made by the trephine in primary or secondary tube placement. It is more useful for tube replacement.

Suppliers

Jones tubes: Gunter Weiss Scientific Glass Blowing Co., 14790 SW Downing Ct. Beaverton, Oregon 97006, USA. UK distributors are Altomed and John Weiss.

K-wires: MicroAire Surgical Instruments, 1641 Edich Drive, Charlottesville, VA 22911 USA.

Bibliography

Boboridis, K. and Olver, J. M. (2000). Endoscopic endonasal assistance with Jones lacrimal bypass tubes. *Ophthal. Surg. Lasers.*, 31, 43–8.

Jones, B. R. (1960). The surgical care of obstruction in the lacrimal canaliculus. *Trans. Ophthal. Soc. UK.*, 80, 343.

Jones, L. T. (1962). The cure of epiphora due to canalicular disorders, trauma and surgical failures on the lacrimal passages. *Trans. Am. Acad. Ophthalmol. Otolaryngol.*, 66, 506–24.

Jones, L. T. (1965). Conjunctivadacryocystorhinostomy. *Am. J. Ophthalmol.*, 59, 773–83.

Jordan, D. R., Nerad, J. A. and Tse, D. T. (1990). The pigtail probe, revisited. *Ophthalmology*, 97, 512–19.

Linberg, J. V. and Moore, C. A. (1988). Symptoms of canalicular obstruction. *Ophthalmology*, 95, 1077–9.

Reifler, D. M. (1991). Management of canalicular laceration. *Surv. Ophthalmol.*, 36, 113–32.

Rose, G. E. and Welham, R. A. N. (1991). Jones' lacrimal canalicular bypass tubes: twenty-five years experience. *Eye*, 5, 13–19.

Smit, T. J. and Mourits, M. (1999). Monocanalicular lesions: to reconstruct or not. *Ophthalmology*, 106, 1310–12.

Trotter, W. L. and Meyer, D. R. (2000). Endoscopic conjunctivodacryocystorhinostomy with Jones tube placement. *Ophthalmology*, 107, 1206–9.

Wearne, M. J., Beigi, B., Davis, G. and Rose, G. E. (1999). Retrograde intubation DCR for proximal and midcanalicular obstruction. *Ophthalmology*, 106, 2325–9.

Welham, R. A. N. (1982). The immediate management of injuries to the lacrimal drainage system. *Trans. Ophthal. Soc. UK.*, 102, 216–17.

Williams, R., Ilsar, M. and Welham, R. A. N. (1985). Lacrimal canalicular papillomatosis. *Br. J. Ophthalmol.*, 69, 464–7.

Yazici, B. and Yazici, Z. (2000). Frequency of the common canaliculus. A radiological study. *Arch. Ophthalmol.*, 118, 1381–5.

CHAPTER 7

Eyelid Surgery

A watering eye is often the result of lower eyelid malposition (ectropion and entropion) or dysfunction (facial palsy and Lax Eyelid Syndrome). In this chapter, the basic surgical techniques for the correction of ectropion and entropion are summarized. Since oculoplastic surgery is well covered in other texts, this is a brief review of useful procedures.

For eyelid anatomy, see Chapter 1; for eyelid assessment, see Chapter 3.

Ectropion

Definition

The eyelid margin is turned away from the eye surface.

Watering

Epiphora is due to reduced tear outflow (punctal stenosis, eyelid malposition, ineffective orbicularis). Hypersecretion occurs from conjunctival irritation. There is coexistent nasolacrimal duct stenosis in some cases.

Ectropion surgery

This depends on the type of ectropion (see Table 7.1).

Table 7.1 Ectropion surgery

Type of ectropion	Surgical options
Involutional	1. Retropunctal cautery 2. Lateral tarsal strip (LTS) and medial spindle (MS) 3. Lazy T (horizontal shortening with adjacent MS) 4. LTS + reattachment of lower lid retractors ± medial canthal tendon stabilization
Paralytic	1. LTS 2. Augmented LTS ± Lee medial canthoplasty (paracanalicular orbicularis to orbicularis) ± sub-orbicularis oculi fat (SOOF) lift ± hard palate mucosal graft
Cicatricial	1. Full thickness skin-orbicularis transposition flap from upper to lower eyelid 2. Full thickness skin graft 3. SOOF lift 4. Z plasty ± horizontal shortening by LTS or full thickness wedge excision
Mechanical	Excise tumour and reconstruct eyelid ± horizontal shorten

Medial spindle (MS) = tarso-conjunctival diamond excision.
For SOOF lift, see Paralytic ectropion.

Practice point: Do not do an isolated MS (tarso-conjunctival diamond excision) without horizontal shortening. It is rarely adequate, and usually reveals horizontal laxity.

Involutional ectropion

Aetiology

There is horizontal lower eyelid laxity, affecting the tarsal plate and the lateral ± medial canthal tendons. The retractors may also be attenuated ('atrophic') or ineffective. There is often anterior lamella shortening, either from actinic changes (sun-damaged skin) or chronic watering. Involutional ectropion is a progressive disorder, starting with punctal ectropion and then involving the rest of the eyelid.

Choice of surgery

1. Very mild punctal ectropion *without* horizontal eyelid laxity – less than 4–5 mm from the globe on pinch test (for how to do the pinch test, see Chapter 3, Assessment of involutional ectropion): retropunctal cautery (Figure 7.1).

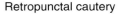

Retropunctal cautery

a
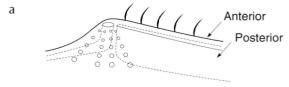
Anterior

Posterior

b　Inverts punctum
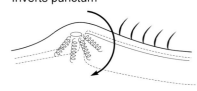

Figure 7.1

Diagrams showing pattern of retropunctal cautery for mild punctal ectropion without horizontal eyelid laxity.

2. All other involutional ectropion:
    - *Primary surgery.* Lateral tarsal strip and medial spindle (LTS + MS). The MS is the tarso-conjunctival diamond excision. Use local anaesthesia. If there is complete tarsal eversion, reattachment of the lower lid retractors via a conjunctival sub-tarsal incision combined with horizontal shortening may be required. If there is anterior lamella shortening (cicatricial element), add tissue appropriately or lift cheek/lower eyelid with a sub-orbicularis oculi fat (SOOF) lift (see Paralytic ectropion). Medial canthal tendon stabilization may be required if there is displacement of the punctum at rest or on the lateral distraction test equivalent to Grade 4 (for how to grade medial canthal tendon laxity, see Chapter 3, Assessment of involutional ectropion).
    - *Redo surgery.* If an initial lateral tarsal strip and medial spindle has failed, horizontal eyelid shortening with repeat medial spindle is recommended. This 'Lazy T' procedure, done under local anaesthesia, is particularly useful where there is medial ectropion with inflamed conjunctiva. The 'Lazy T' combines full thickness eyelid wedge excision with an adjacent MS (tarso-conjunctival diamond excision). After surgery, the cuts on the conjunctival surface resemble a 'T' on its side, hence it is called 'Lazy T' (see Figure 7.6).

TIP

Mimic the effect of surgery digitally, by tightening the eyelid laterally and inverting the margin (LTS and MS, or LTS and retractor reattachment), or pinch the eyelid medially (Lazy T) to confirm that the surgery will work.

Practice point: Ectropion is less marked when the patient lies flat, and more noticeable when the patient is sitting or standing.

Non-surgical management

Pre-treat inflamed ectropion eyelids with steroid-antibiotic ointment twice daily for 2 weeks prior to surgery.

Surgical techniques

Lateral tarsal strip (LTS)

The lower eyelid is shortened horizontally at the lateral canthus by creating a strip of tissue from the lateral end of the tarsal plate, which is tucked inside the lateral orbital rim. This shortens and elevates the lower eyelid, giving it a youthful appearance, and maintains a sharp lateral canthal angle. The strip is made as follows (Figures 7.2, 7.3):

1. Do lateral canthotomy (horizontal cut at the lateral canthus which divides the inferior crus of the lateral canthal tendon).
2. Do lateral cantholysis (vertical cut within the lateral eyelid which divides the orbital septum and vertical part of the inferior crus from the lateral orbital rim).
3. Remove the lateral lashes, a small slither of anterior lamella skin and orbicularis, and the posterior conjunctiva.
4. Attach a permanent 5.0 suture (e.g. Ethibond or Prolene), which is passed through the orbital rim periosteum from posterior to anterior, and the eyelid tightened.
5. Take great care in closing the wound in layers (orbicularis then skin), to prevent potential complications of infection and granuloma formation around the deep suture.

A medial spindle is done simultaneously, and this must be completed *before* tightening the lateral tarsal strip.

Medial spindle

A small, diamond-shaped section of posterior lamella just below the punctum is excised and sutured closed, in order to invert the punctum. The closing suture tries to catch the medial edge of the inferior retractors, to assist inverting the medial eyelid on blinking. The excised tissue is usually the conjunctiva overlying the lower medial tarsal plate; hence it is called tarso-conjunctival diamond excision. Deeper tissue can be excised if necessary, including the orbital septum and upper edge of retractors. It is called a medial spindle because of its shape when cut out with curved conjunctival scissors. It is also called a medial kite when it is made longer lateral to the punctum, to increase its effect. If a medial spindle or diamond shape is excised, one inverting suture is

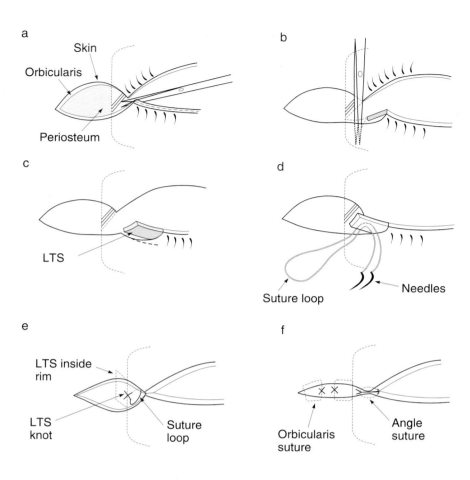

a

Skin
Orbicularis
Periosteum

b

c

LTS

d

Suture loop

Needles

e

LTS inside rim
LTS knot
Suture loop

f

Orbicularis suture
Angle suture

Figure 7.2

Diagrams showing steps for lateral tarsal strip.

a) Skin orbicularis incision down to lateral orbital rim periosteum and lateral canthotomy.

b) Lateral cantholysis to release lower eyelid.

c) Lateral tarsal strip created by excising a small strip of skin, eyelashes and orbicularis from the anterior surface, excising the mucocutaneous junction and the conjunctiva on the posterior surface.

d) A double-ended 5.0 Ethibond suture is placed on the strip close to the medial end. The suture ends should emerge from the anterior surface of the strip so that the lateral length of the strip can be tucked inside the orbital rim.

e) The knot is secured on the anterior orbital rim.

f) The lateral canthal angle is closed with a buried 6.0 Vicryl suture, the orbicularis is closed with two 6.0 Vicryl purse string sutures. The skin is then closed with 8.0 Vicryl interrupted sutures.

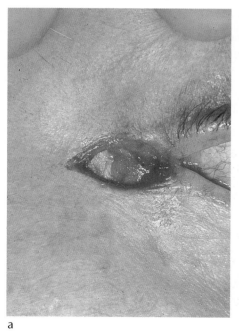

a

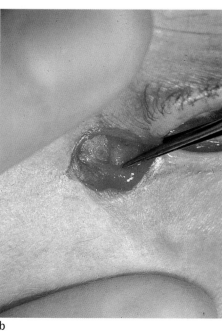

b

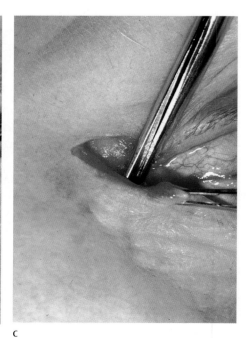

c

Figure 7.3 Right lateral tarsal strip.

a) Skin orbicularis incision down to lateral orbital rim.
b) Lateral canthotomy with straight blunt scissors. The lower limb of the lateral canthal tendon is divided.
c) Lateral cantholysis with straight, sharp scissors.

continued

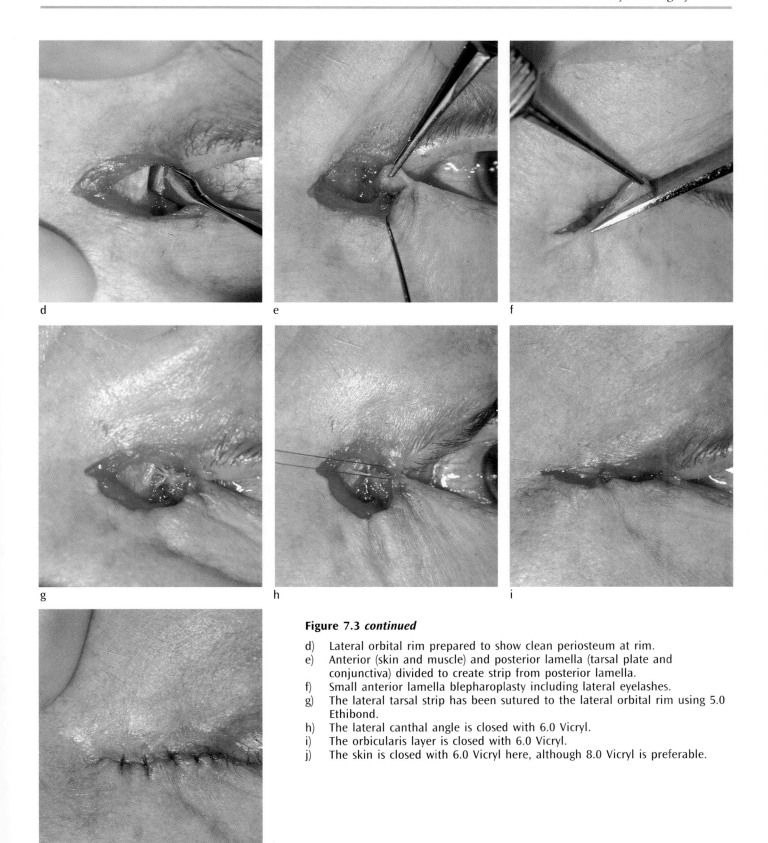

Figure 7.3 *continued*

d) Lateral orbital rim prepared to show clean periosteum at rim.
e) Anterior (skin and muscle) and posterior lamella (tarsal plate and conjunctiva) divided to create strip from posterior lamella.
f) Small anterior lamella blepharoplasty including lateral eyelashes.
g) The lateral tarsal strip has been sutured to the lateral orbital rim using 5.0 Ethibond.
h) The lateral canthal angle is closed with 6.0 Vicryl.
i) The orbicularis layer is closed with 6.0 Vicryl.
j) The skin is closed with 6.0 Vicryl here, although 8.0 Vicryl is preferable.

a

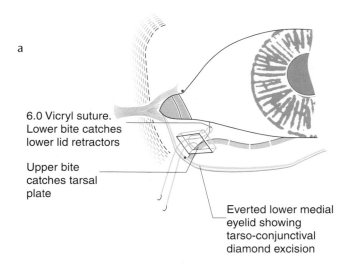

6.0 Vicryl suture.
Lower bite catches
lower lid retractors

Upper bite
catches tarsal
plate

Everted lower medial
eyelid showing
tarso-conjunctival
diamond excision

b

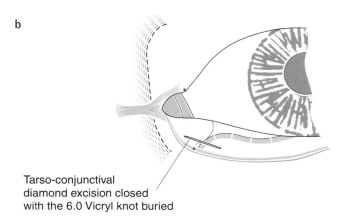

Tarso-conjunctival
diamond excision closed
with the 6.0 Vicryl knot buried

Figure 7.4

Diagrams showing the medial spindle suture.
a)   Placement of the 6.0 Vicryl buried suture to close the
     medial spindle (diamond-shaped tarso-conjunctival
     excision).
b)   Appearance when suture is tightened and secured.

required to close the spindle/diamond, but if a kite
shape is excised, place two inverting sutures (Figures 7.4,
7.5).

'Lazy T'

This combines full thickness horizontal eyelid
shortening with an adjacent medial spindle (Figure 7.6).

Medial canthal tendon stabilization

The medial canthal tendon laxity is corrected by
plicating or stabilizing the anterior limb of the medial
canthal tendon. This is done by a permanent suture
placed between the medial inferior tarsal edge and the
upper part of the medial canthal tendon and periosteum
on the ascending frontal process of the maxilla. It is
easiest to use a double-armed Prolene non-absorbable
suture (e.g. 6/0 or 5/0 Prolene). The tarsal plate is either
reached via the skin (transcutaneous) or the medial
spindle (transconjunctival).

Severe MCT laxity affecting the posterior limb (e.g. in
trauma) is repaired by a posterior fixation suture to the
posterior lacrimal crest from the medial end of the tarsal
plate. The technique involves a retro-plical incision
towards the posterior lacrimal crest (Figures 7.7–7.9).

Post-operative management – ectropion

The patient is instructed to insert topical antibiotic
drops ×4 for 2 weeks and advised *not* to pull the lower
eyelid down whilst inserting the drops.

Follow-up – ectropion

The LTS + MS patient need not be seen for up to 3
weeks, as the skin sutures do not need removing. The
Lazy T patient requires more intensive follow-up, for
removal of the skin sutures 1 week after surgery and the
lid margin sutures 2 weeks after surgery. Subsequent
follow-up for both procedures is 3 and 6 months after
surgery, remembering to ask about the initial symptoms
of watering (the reason the surgery was done). If MCT
stabilization was done, review at 1 week and 1, 3 and 6
months.

Complications following ectropion surgery

1.   LTS:
     ● Lateral orbital rim tenderness in up to 25 per
       cent of patients for about 2 months after
       surgery. Warn patients before surgery to expect
       this.
     ● Wound dehiscence is rare. The lateral canthal
       angle suture helps hold the lower eyelid in place.

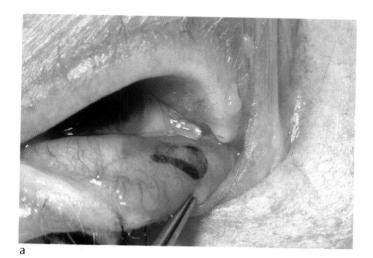

a

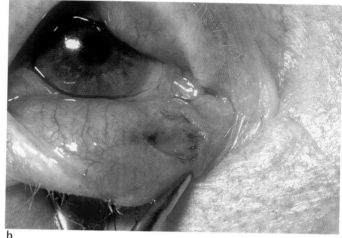

b

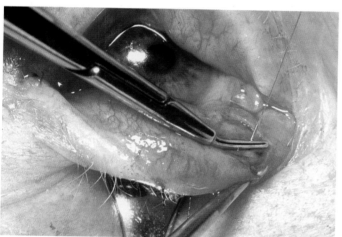

c

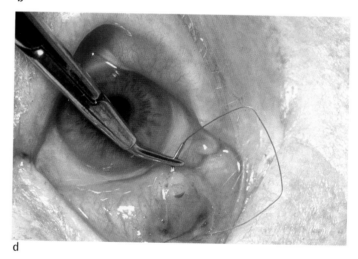

d

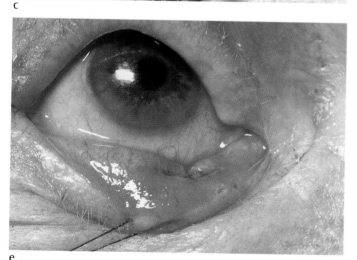

e

Figure 7.5

Per-operative pictures of a medial spindle (MS).

a) A 6.0 black silk traction suture is placed through the grey line and the lower eyelid is everted over a Desmarre's retractor. A Nettleship dilator or Bowman probe is placed in the lower punctum to localize it. The medial spindle (MS) or diamond of tarso-conjunctiva is outlined.

b) The conjunctiva is excised (deeper tissue can be excised in severe ectropion). The apex is approximately 2 mm below the punctum. The bed of the MS consists of the tarsal plate superior and lower eyelid retractors inferior. The marginal artery is found at the lower border of the tarsal plate and may bleed; it is easily cauterized with bipolar cautery.

c) The MS is closed with a single 6.0 Vicryl suture with a half-circle needle. The suture makes a small bite of the tarsal plate at the apex of the MS going from inside the spindle towards the apex, not including the conjunctiva.

d) A bite is made into the lower apex of the spindle from inferior to superior, catching the lower eyelid retractors. Both suture ends are then pulled out laterally, keeping the loop medial, and tightened in the line of the wound.

e) The suture is secured and trimmed short. Subsequently the LTS is done.

Lazy T

a

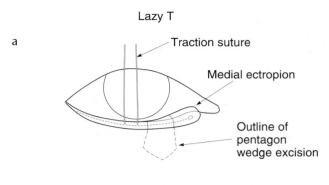

Traction suture

Medial ectropion

Outline of pentagon wedge excision

b

Eyelid everted

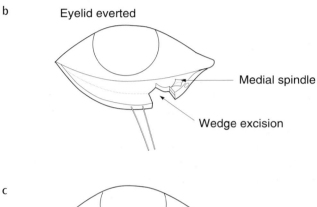

Medial spindle

Wedge excision

c

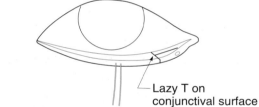

Lazy T on conjunctival surface

Figure 7.6

Diagrams showing Lazy-T procedure.
a) The amount of horizontal shortening required is marked.
b) Full thickness horizontal wedge excision and medial spindle (tarso-conjunctival diamond excision).
c) Appearance after repair.

- Suture extrusion, granuloma or infection is a risk if the permanent non-absorbable suture is not well buried within the tissue.
2. MS:
   - Undercorrection may occur if the inverting suture is not well placed and tightened.
   - Early mucous discharge is associated with absorbable sutures.
3. Lazy T:
   - Wound infection and dehiscence.
   - Lid margin notch.

a

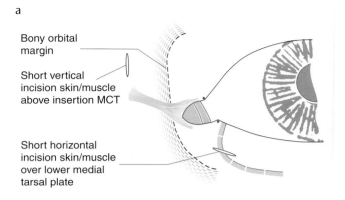

Bony orbital margin

Short vertical incision skin/muscle above insertion MCT

Short horizontal incision skin/muscle over lower medial tarsal plate

b

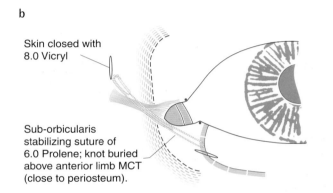

Skin closed with 8.0 Vicryl

Sub-orbicularis stabilizing suture of 6.0 Prolene; knot buried above anterior limb MCT (close to periosteum).

Figure 7.7

Transcutaneous medial canthal tendon stabilization.
a) Two small incisions.
b) Buried permanent suture between medial-inferior edge of lower tarsal plate and periosteum on ascending process maxilla above the MCT.

- Reduced horizontal palpebral aperture.
4. MCT stabilization:
   - Risk of suture extrusion or lump on maxilla above the MCT where non-absorbable suture knot is buried.
   - Risk of recurrent laxity from suture cheese-wiring and becoming slack.

Paralytic ectropion

Aetiology

Orbicularis weakness causes lacrimal pump dysfunction. There is also lower eyelid sag or overt ectropion, giving a

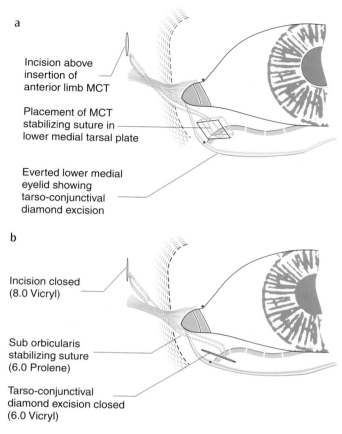

a

Incision above insertion of anterior limb MCT

Placement of MCT stabilizing suture in lower medial tarsal plate

Everted lower medial eyelid showing tarso-conjunctival diamond excision

b

Incision closed (8.0 Vicryl)

Sub orbicularis stabilizing suture (6.0 Prolene)

Tarso-conjunctival diamond excision closed (6.0 Vicryl)

Figure 7.8

Transconjunctival (via medial spindle) approach medial canthal tendon stabilization.
a)   The permanent stabilization suture is first passed through the inferior-medial edge of the lower tarsal plate then fed through the tissue to above the MCT.
b)   The medial spindle is closed in the standard fashion.

widened palpebral aperture and lagophthalmos. The blink excursion is reduced. The eye may water (combined epiphora and hypersecretion) or feel dry. With time, there is increasing lower eyelid laxity, orbicularis atrophy and mid-face ptosis. Corneal exposure is exacerbated when there is coexistent corneal anaesthesia.

Non-surgical management

- Treatment with lubricant drops (e.g. guttae hypromellose or carboners) and paraffin eye ointment or taping the eyelid shut at night to reduce the risk of exposure keratitis. Punctal occlusive plugs

can help reduce the need for frequent lubricants in selected patients.
- Use Botulinum toxin A chemodenervation of the levator palpebrae superioris for temporary ptosis to treat exposure keratitis, especially if the cornea is neuropathic. The ptosis reverses spontaneously after 3 months. Spread of toxin to the superior rectus may occur, but is rarely troublesome since the visual axis is covered by the upper eyelid. Toxin spread is reduced by injection into the supra-tarsal subconjunctival space where a smaller dose is used.

Choice of surgery

1.   Lateral tarsorrhaphy is not recommended, as it fails to shorten the lower eyelid enough and gives a blinkering effect where the patient loses peripheral visual field.
2.   Do a simple LTS to elevate and tighten the lower lid. It can be reversed if there is recovery of function, without permanent disfigurement.
3.   If the palsy is severe or longstanding, do an augmented LTS. This allows differential shortening of the upper and lower eyelid (greater lower eyelid shortening) and enables the strip to be placed much higher up on the lateral orbital rim. It can be combined with the insertion of a hard palate mucosal graft or Medpor® lid implant for extra lower eyelid lift.
4.   Both the LTS and augmented LTS can be combined with a SOOF lift if there is an associated mid-face ptosis with prominent palpebral-malar fold.
5.   If the medial palpebral aperture is widened, a Lee medial canthoplasty is used to narrow the vertical palpebral aperture medial to the puncta by joining the orbicularis above and below the canaliculi.
6.   Use upper eyelid gold weight to improve blink excursion.
7.   If the patient still requires a lot of topical lubricants after the above surgery, consider lower punctal silicone plugs (e.g. FCI punctal occlusive silicone plugs). If the cornea is anaesthetic, use both lower and upper punctal plugs.

Practice point: If the cornea is anaesthetic, surgery must reduce the vertical palpebral aperture to less than that of the normal side and plugs should be considered to reduce the frequency of lubricants.

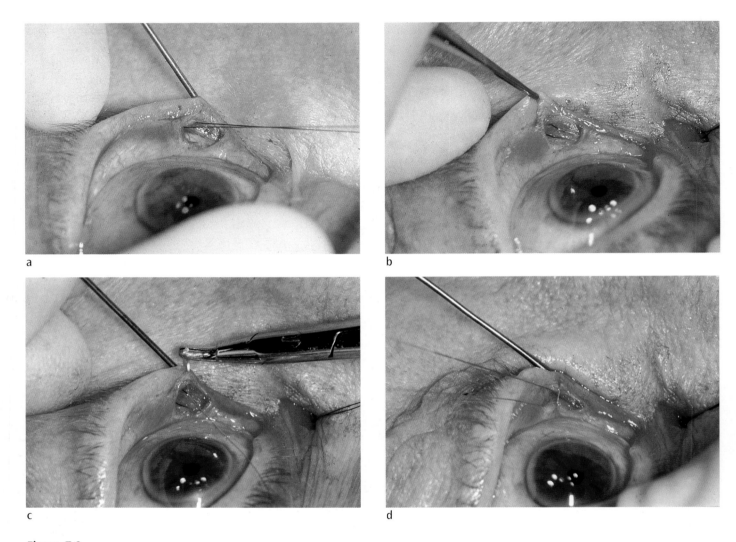

Figure 7.9

Transconjunctival approach (medial spindle) medial canthal tendon stabilization suture.
a) The 6.0 Prolene suture is attached to the lower medial border of the inferior tarsal plate.
b) The Prolene suture has been passed through the tissue to emerge just above the medial canthal tendon insertion on the ascending process of the maxilla.
c) The tip of the 6.0 Vicryl needle is being pulled out at the apex of the spindle just below the punctum. Note that the Prolene suture is not caught in the Vicryl suture.
d) The lower Vicryl bite at the inferior apex of the spindle has been made and both ends are pulled laterally to close the spindle. The suture is then secured in a standard way. This buries the Prolene suture.

Augmented LTS

A long lateral tarsal strip is taken up through the upper eyelid margin and sutured to the outside of the lateral orbital rim in its upper third, under local anaesthesia. For a good result there should be an initial over-correction, with the lower lid lifted quite high and sloping supero-laterally.

If a hard palate mucosal graft is added, do under general anaesthesia. Special nasal intubation assists access for harvesting the graft, and this may need prior discussion with the anaesthetist (Figures 7.10, 7.11).

Augmented LTS

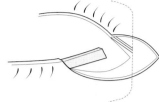

a

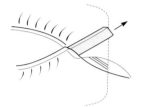

b

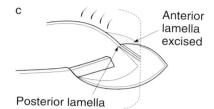

c

Anterior lamella excised

Posterior lamella

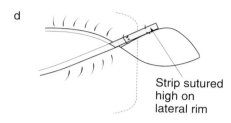

d

Strip sutured high on lateral rim

Figure 7.10

Diagram showing the augmented lateral tarsal strip.

a) A long lower eyelid strip has been fashioned.

b) The lower lid strip is directed upwards and laterally to the superior-lateral orbital rim to decide how much upper eyelid anterior lamella must be excised.

c) The upper eyelid is split laterally into anterior and posterior lamellae for a short distance, and an anterior lamella slither (with eyelashes) is excised.

d) The new lateral canthal angle is sutured and then the augmented lateral tarsal strip secured to the outside of the rim at the highest point it will reach. Standard two-layer closure follows.

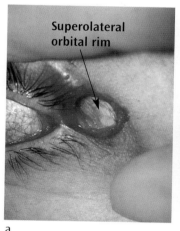

Superolateral orbital rim

a

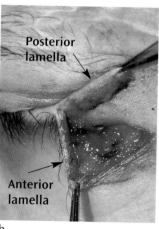

Posterior lamella

Anterior lamella

b

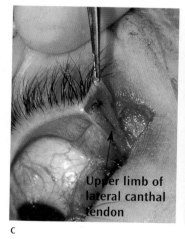

Upper limb of lateral canthal tendon

c

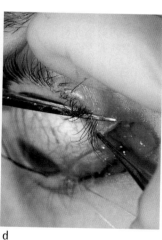

d

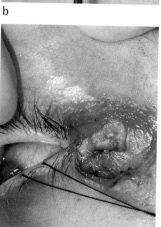

e

f

Figure 7.11

Left augmented lateral tarsal strip.

a) Lateral canthal skin orbicularis incision to the supero-lateral orbital rim.

b) A long strip is prepared by dividing the anterior and posterior lamellae. The strip is shown here directed supero-lateral, overlapping the upper lateral eyelid.

c) The upper eyelid anterior and posterior lamellae are split, without detaching the upper limb of the lateral canthal tendon (arrow).

d) A small slither of anterior lamella, including the lateral lashes, is excised.

e) Left lateral canthus showing differential shortening of the lower and upper anterior lamella. The LTS is long and has a 5.0 Ethibond suture (white) attached close to its medial end. The black suture seen far left is the lid traction suture.

f) The long LTS is sutured to the supero-lateral orbital rim. Additional bites of periosteum are taken to secure the strip flat at its lateral tip.

a

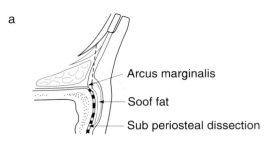

Arcus marginalis

Soof fat

Sub periosteal dissection

b

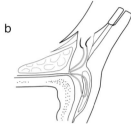

Figure 7.12

Diagram showing position of SOOF fat and lift.
a) Conjunctival approaches.
b) Sutures from undersurface SOOF to arcus marginalis and to superficial temporal fascia/periosteum at lateral orbital rim.

SOOF lift

The sub-orbicularis oculi fat pad and overlying skin and muscle is elevated and hence the lower eyelid raised. Surgery is under general anaesthesia, via a swinging eyelid flap, through a transconjunctival subperiosteal approach, which combines eyelid shortening with SOOF elevation. Periosteal adhesions over the maxilla down to the gingiva are freed, preserving the infra-orbital nerve. The SOOF is re-attached to the arcus marginalis on the inferior orbital rim and to the superficial temporal fascia on the lateral orbital rim (Figure 7.12). This procedure can also be done with the help of an endoscope via a Caldwell Luc gingival incision (above the incisor tooth).

Lee medial canthoplasty

A paracanalicular skin incision is made medial to the puncta (with Bowman probes *in situ*) and the para-canalicular orbicularis is sutured using two 6/0 non-absorbable mattress sutures to reduce the medial vertical palpebral aperture.

Post-operative management

The post-operative management of the augmented LTS is the same as for the simple LTS. If there is excessive swelling, use a non-steroidal anti-inflammatory orally after day 4 (prior to that may cause bleeding).

Hard palate mucosal grafts and SOOF lift patients require post-operative systemic antibiotics for 1 week, and non-steroidal anti-inflammatory tablets for up to 3 weeks (starting day 4 or 5 post-operatively), as well as topical guttae chloromycetin and dexamethasone ×4 for 3 weeks.

Follow-up

The follow-up for the augmented LTS is similar to that for the LTS.

The hard palate mucosal grafts and SOOF lift patients should be seen at 1, 2 and 4 weeks after surgery, then at 3 and 6 months.

Complications

1. Augmented LTS:
    ● Lateral orbital rim tenderness.
2. SOOF lift:
    ● Chemosis and eyelid swelling
    ● Cellulitis.
3. Lee medial canthoplasty:
    ● Re-opening/stretch
    ● Conceals puncta
    ● Watering is worse.

Entropion

Definition

Eyelid rotation or inturning towards the globe.

Practice point: Trichiasis is eyelashes growing towards the ocular surface, without eyelid margin inturning (entropion).

Watering

Contact of the eyelid skin and lashes with the surface of eye causes irritation, discomfort, pain, redness and corneal epithelial breakdown. There is reflex hypersecretion and some orbicularis dysfunction (lacrimal pump failure) due to the preseptal orbicularis overriding the pretarsal orbicularis.

Entropion surgery

This depends on the type of entropion (see Table 7.2).

> **TIP**
>
> *In the assessment of entropion, evaluate the horizontal and vertical (retractors) laxity and look for posterior lamella shortening.*

Resume eyelid assessment

1. To assess horizontal laxity, measure the horizontal eyelid laxity (HEL) and medial canthal tendon laxity (MCT grade).

Table 7.2 Entropion surgery

Type of entropion	Surgical options
Involutional	1. Quickert-Rathbun everting sutures 2. Lateral tarsal strip (LTS) and four Quickert everting sutures 3. LTS and Jones retractor plication via partial thickness horizontal eyelid incision 4. LTS and diagonal tightening of both retractors and orbital septum 5. Quickert procedure: horizontal shortening by full thickness wedge excision plus retractor plication
Cicatricial	1. LTS and hard palate mucosal graft 2. Jones retractor plication via partial thickness eyelid incision plus full thickness horizontal eyelid incision 3. Lamella split and cryotherapy to anterior lamella 4. Extended Hotz procedure (ellipse skin and muscle excision)
Congenital (epiblepharon)	Hotz procedure (ellipse of medial anterior lamella, skin and muscle excised)

2. To assess vertical laxity, observe fat prolapse (orbital septal thinning) and look at the sub-tarsal conjunctiva for retractor dehiscence.
3. To assess posterior lamella shortening, examine the tarsal conjunctiva with a green light on the slit-lamp to help see scarring and measure the fornix depth.

Involutional entropion

Aetiology

Horizontal and vertical (lower eyelid retractors) laxity ± enophthalmos ± orbital fat prolapse from septal thinning.

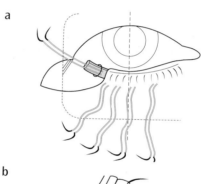

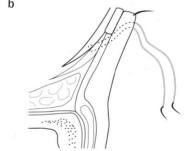

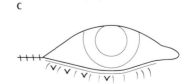

Figure 7.13

a) Prepared LTS and four pre-placed everting sutures for involutional entropion correction. Do not place everting sutures too medial.
b) Everting sutures.
c) Eyelid appearance at end of operation.

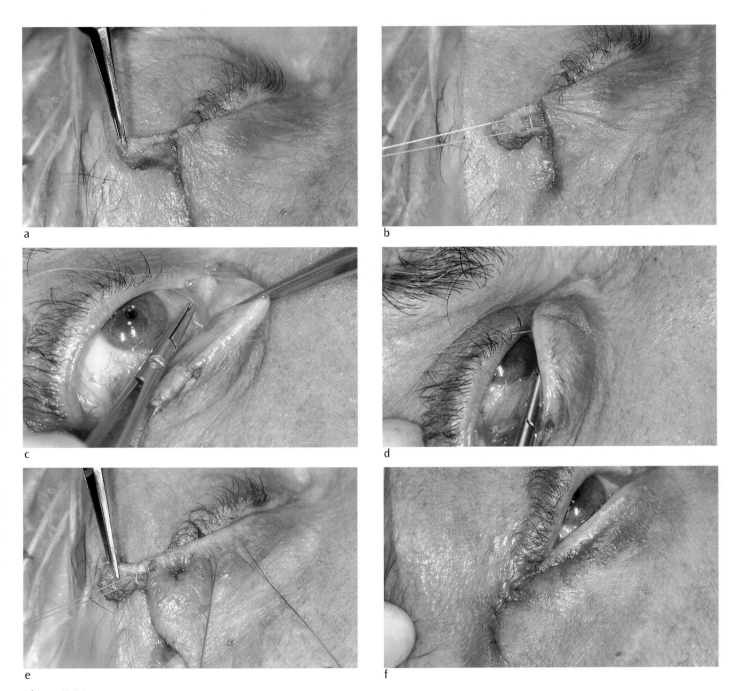

a

b

c

d

e

f

Figure 7.14

Per-operative pictures of the LTS and everting sutures for involutional entropion.

a) Standard LTS.

b) 5.0 Ethibond suture attached to strip but not secured to the lateral orbital rim until after all the everting sutures have been placed.

c) Medial 6.0 Vicryl (double-ended, half-circle needle) everting suture passed from conjunctival surface low down to skin surface, just below the eyelashes.

d) Tip of everting suture emerging. Both ends are passed from the conjunctiva (low) to the skin (high) and placed on a bulldog clip. Up to three further sutures are similarly placed.

e) The everting sutures are tightened here before the LTS is attached (it is only sometimes easier to tighten them after the LTS has been secured).

f) All everting sutures have been tied and trimmed and the LTS secured and closed in the standard way. 6.0 Vicryl sutures have been used on the skin, since there is plenty of this suture available!

Practice point: Entropion is worse lying flat, when the orbital soft tissues sink back into the socket, giving a relative enophthalmos.

Non-surgical management

Lower eyelid taping to evert the lid and topical lubricants provide temporary symptomatic relief.

Botulinum toxin A injected into the preseptal orbicularis (10–15 units Dysport®, Ipsen, or 3–4 units Botox®, Allergan), just lateral to the mid-point reverses the entropion for up to 4 months. This is particularly useful if the patient is bed-bound or unsuitable for surgery, and the procedure can be repeated. Side effects (< 5 per cent) include lower facial drop and diplopia from the spread of toxin, usually dose related.

Choice of surgery

Both the horizontal and vertical laxity must be addressed. Simple Quickert everting sutures are reported as effective in up to 75 per cent of eyelids for over 18 months, but do not correct horizontal laxity. It is best to restrict their use to eyelids without horizontal eyelid laxity, or to combine them with eyelid shortening.

The Quickert procedure is ideal, as it addresses both horizontal and vertical laxity, but it requires more intensive post-operative management than the LTS and everting sutures or diagonal tightening of the retractors and orbital septum, which are both via a small lateral canthal incision. A combination of the LTS and lower lid retractor plication (Jones procedure) is popular, but is more invasive than the LTS and everting sutures and has a greater post-operative morbidity due to suture-related problems.

Surgical technique

LTS and four everting sutures

A standard LTS is prepared and the 5/0 non-absorbable suture (e.g. Ethibond) is placed on a bulldog clip. Four 6/0 non-absorbable (e.g. Vicryl) everting sutures are placed. The LTS is sutured inside the lateral orbital rim.

The lateral canthotomy wound is closed in the standard fashion. The everting sutures are tied firmly (Figures 7.13, 7.14).

Post-operative management

The patient is instructed to insert topical antibiotic drops ×4 for up to 2 weeks, without pulling the eyelid down. The everting sutures must not be removed, but are left to hydrolyse over the next 6–10 weeks. Vicryl is less inflammatory than catgut, which can produce an aggressive and unpredictable local reaction.

Follow-up

The patient is seen once between 1 and 3 weeks after surgery, then at 3, 6 and 12 months. The lateral canthal wound has 8.0 or 6.0 Vicryl sutures, which do not require removing.

Complications

1. Those of the LTS (see above).
2. Rarely, everting suture knot inflammation.
3. Warn the patient that the everting sutures can be felt for a few weeks as 'bristles' below the lash line. In practice, some of the everting sutures bury in.

Bibliography

Blaydon, S. M. and Neuhaus, R. W. (2000). Entropion repair: anatomical approach. In: *New Orleans Academy of Ophthalmology. Current Concepts in Aesthetic and Reconstructive Oculoplastic Surgery* (C. L. Fry, ed.), pp. 181–192. Kugler Publications.

Collin, J. R. and Rathbun, J. F. (1978). Involutional entropion: a review with evaluation of a procedure. *Arch. Ophthalmol.* 96, 1058–64.

Manners, R. (1995). Surgical repair of medial ectropion. *Eye*, 9, 365–7.

Olver, J. M. (1998). Surgical tips on the lateral tarsal strip. *Eye*, **12**, 1007–12.

Olver, J. (2000). Raising the SOOF, its role in chronic facial palsy. *Br. J. Ophthalmol.*, **84**, 1401–6.

Olver, J. M. and Barnes, J. (2000). Effective small incision surgery for involutional lower lid entropion. *Ophthalmology*, **107**, 1982–8.

Quickert, M. H. and Rathbun, J. E. (1971). Suture repair of entropion. *Arch. Ophthalmol.*, 85(3), 304–5.

Tse, D. T. (1985). Surgical correction of punctal malposition. *Am. J. Ophthalmol.*, **100**, 339–41.

Van den Bosch, W. A. and Lemij, H. G. (1994). The lax eyelid syndrome. *Br. J. Ophthalmol.*, **78**, 666–70.

CHAPTER 8

Recent Advances in Lacrimal Surgery

In this chapter more recent advances, some of which are still being evaluated, are summarized:

1. Botulinum toxin – a treatment for crocodile tears
2. Punctal plugs in facial palsy
3. Transcanalicular laser canaliculoplasty and dacryocystorhinostomy
4. Adult nasolacrimal duct intubation
5. Balloon catheter dilation of the nasolacrimal duct (dacryoplasty)
6. Nasolacrimal duct stents.

Botulinum toxin – a treatment for crocodile tears

Injection of 15–20 units Dysport® (Ipsen Ltd, Maidenhead, Berkshire, UK) or 3–4 units BOTOX® (Allergan) directly into the lacrimal gland, either transcutaneously or transconjunctivally, reduces crocodile tears in patients with VIIth nerve palsy. Injections must be repeated every 3–4 months. Occasional side effects include ptosis and diplopia from the spread of toxin. Posterior dacryectomy is the surgical alternative.

Punctal plugs in facial palsy

Silicone punctal plugs to occlude the lower ± upper puncta increase tear retention in cases of severe dry eye (e.g. Sjögren's Syndrome, Stevens–Johnson Syndrome).

Silicone plugs are also used in longstanding facial palsy with residual exposure keratitis requiring frequent topical lubricants after eyelid surgery, especially when there is a neuropathic cornea. These are placed after palpebral and malar surgery has been completed. The decision to insert them is based on the patient's symptoms and lubricant regime, the appearance of the tear film, and corneal and interpalpebral fluorescein punctal stain.

Should there be a trial of collagen plugs?

Silicone plugs are permanent yet also reversible, as they are easily removed with forceps at the slit-lamp. It is not necessary to do a trial of collagen plugs, which only last a few hours, therefore often failing to predict the effect of silicone plugs and necessitating an extra patient visit.

How to insert silicone punctal plugs

The plugs are inserted under topical ± local infiltrative anaesthesia, using either the slit-lamp or operating microscope for magnification. The plug is pre-mounted. The most common size is 'Regular'; occasionally a larger size is required, and 0.6, 0.8 and 1.0 mm diameters are in use (Figure 8.1).

1. Dilate the punctum well

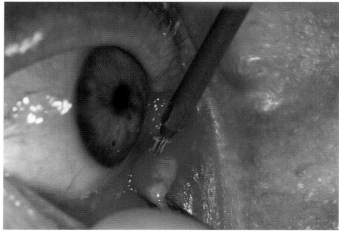

a

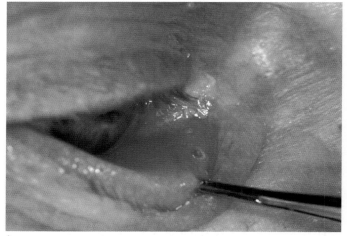

b

Figure 8.1
a) Pre-mounted ready-to-insert punctal plug. The lower punctum has been dilated and plug insertion was difficult, therefore local anaesthetic was injected and the eyelid held in forceps.
b) Plug in place.

2. Keep the eyelid on lateral stretch whilst inserting the plug into the dilated punctum
3. Note that the slope of the head of the plug has an angle with the body, which reflects the slope of the eyelid medial to the punctum
4. If necessary, infiltrate local anaesthesia into the medial eyelid and hold the eyelid margin with forceps at a point lateral to the punctum to facilitate plug insertion.

Post-operative management

No additional topical medication is required. Observe regularly in clinic. Patients reduce the lubricants as they feel appropriate. Insert second plug or remove plugs as indicated.

Complications

Complications include:

- Plug loss (it falls out)
- The plug travelling down canaliculus (may cause canaliculitis)
- Pyogenic granuloma.

The most common complication is plug loss (it falls out). If a good quality and suitable size plug is used and inserted correctly, disappearance into the canaliculus with resultant canaliculitis is extremely rare.

Transcanalicular laser canaliculoplasty and dacryocystorhinostomy

Diagnostic transcanalicular endoscopy reveals the normal and abnormal appearance of the proximal lacrimal system, including the detection of canalicular folds, lacrimal sac dacryoliths, other intra-sac pathology, and bony protrusions. Systems such as the Miniflex from Laserscope use a 0.8 mm outer diameter lacrimal endoscope (Figure 8.2).

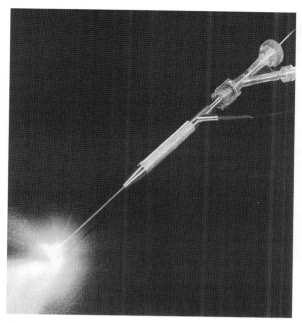

Figure 8.2

Modified lacrimal endoscope with three ports. The laser fibre is inserted via the central port and irrigation through the side port of the two-way tap. The light and camera are attached at the side of the probe. Mueller, K. (2000) Endolacrimal laser assisted lacrimal surgery. *Br. J. Ophthalmol.* With permission from BMJ Publishing Group.

Coupling the mini-endoscope with a laser or micro-drill enables intra-lacrimal system treatment of canalicular folds, stenosis, dacryoliths, bony protrusions and dacryocystorhinostomy (DCR). A xenon light source is used. Either a fine rigid endoscope (0.9–1.3 mm diameter) or flexible endoscope (0.3–0.5 mm diameter) placed inside a rigid Junemann probe (0.7–1.1 mm diameter) is used. An irrigation system is attached. The Miniflex system uses a 1.1 mm outer diameter lacrimal endoscope through which a 200 or 300 μm laser fibre is passed.

Transcanalicular laser-assisted DCR has poor results, which depend on the type of laser and whether the rhinostomy is surgically assisted (30–78 per cent success rate).

Laser canaliculoplasty

Early experience of laser canaliculoplasty using the holmium laser was done without a transcanalicular

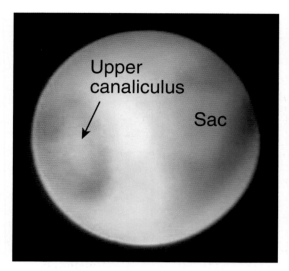

Figure 8.3

Miniflex (Laserscope) view of left inflamed lacrimal sac (right) and opening of upper canaliculus (left) in a patient with an expressible mucocoele.

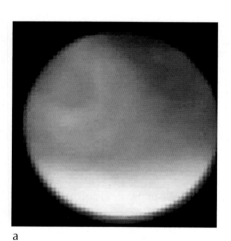

a

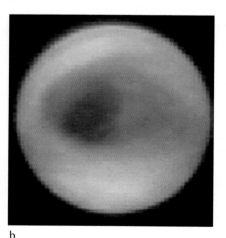

b

Figure 8.4

a)   Intra-canalicular endoscopy. Mini-endoscope view of lower canalicular showing stenosis (with permission, Muellner *et al.*, 2000 and *British Journal of Ophthalmology*).

b)   After opening with laser.

endoscope. The success rates were low; 57 per cent anatomical patency and 43 per cent subjective improvement of epiphora (Dutton and Holck, 1996).

More recent transcanalicular treatment of canalicular obstructions up to 2 mm long uses a mini-endoscope with a microtrephine or erbium : YAG laser, with or without silicone intubation (Figures 8.3, 8.4). The results

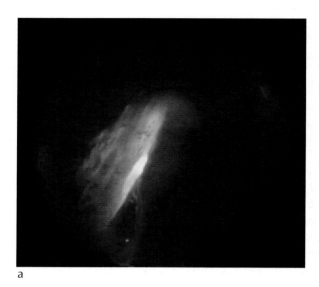

a

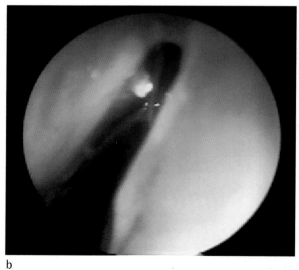

b

Figure 8.5

a)   Transcanalicular KTP laser seen endonasally. Green light is used during laser procedure.

b)   View of laser probe emerging into nose through lacrimal sac mucosa, lacrimal bone and nasal mucosa (with permission, Muellner *et al.*, 2000 and *British Journal of Ophthalmology*).

Table 8.1 Results of transcanalicular laser-assisted DCR

Author/year	Rhinostomy	Type of laser	Type of DCR	Subjective success rate (%)
Piaton, 1994	Laser	Neodymium : YAG	Re-do and primary	75
Dalez, 1996	Laser	Holmium : YAG	Primary	47
Patel, 1997	Laser	Neodymium : YAG	Re-do	46
Rosen, 1997	Laser	Neodymium : YAG	Primary	64
Muellner *et al.*, 2000	Laser and transnasal drill	KTP	Primary	78
Eloy *et al.*, 2000	Laser	Diode	Primary	70 (approx.)

are promising, showing that it is effective in 70–84 per cent of selected cases.

Laser dacryocystorhinostomy

Transcanalicular laser DCR (primary and re-do) using the Nd : YAG or the KTP laser is still being established (Figure 8.5). Several surgeons have given up using the laser for the transcanalicular rhinostomy. In particular, attempts with the holmium : YAG or diode laser have shown poor results and have been abandoned. There is a higher rate of minor complications. Transcanalicular

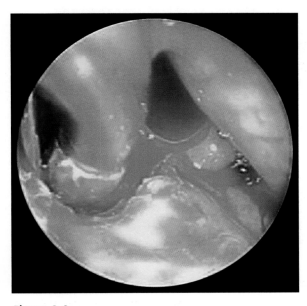

Figure 8.6

Endonasal assistance with micro-drill to increase size of rhinostomy made by endocanalicular KTP laser (with permission, Muellner *et al.*, 2000 and *British Journal of Ophthalmology*).

DCR either uses the laser alone, or the operation is assisted by endonasal surgical instruments (such as a drill) for the rhinostomy, which appears to give better long-term results (Figure 8.6). Silicone intubation is required.

Results of transcanalicular laser-assisted DCR

These are shown in Table 8.1.

KTP laser parameters for transcanalicular DCR:	
Wavelength	532 nm
Power	5–10 W
Delivery service	300, 400 or 600 µm fibre
Mode	Q switch in continuous or 0.5 s repeated pulses (500 ms/1 pps)
Technique	Near contact (coagulates)/contact (cuts)

Another transcanalicular DCR technique uses a microdrill for post-sac stenosis rather than a laser, with all the surgery confined within the lacrimal system.

Transcanalicular laser conjunctivo-DCR and Jones tube placement

Transcanalicular diode laser directs the energy away from the eye, as opposed to towards the eye with the endonasal holmium : YAG laser primary conjunctivo-DCR. The probe must be able to enter a significant portion of canaliculus and be held firmly against the bone to be effective and avoid soft tissue injury at the medial canthus, which is not always possible.

Adult nasolacrimal duct intubation

Adult nasolacrimal duct intubation was popular in the 1970s, and the concept is being revisited as a means of avoiding a DCR for canalicular obstruction (where the nasolacrimal duct may be normal) and for partial or complete nasolacrimal duct stenosis. The availability of the nasal endoscope has made retrieval of tubes in the inferior meatus very easy. The following types of intubation are used:

1. Crawford tubes with attached long flexible metal bodkins (Chapter 4, Figure 4.16)
2. Ritleng tubes with a specially designed introducer
3. Double bicanalicular Hausler tubes (Figure 8.7) – these are also used for DCR
4. Nunchaku tubes, which are inserted with two introducers and have no intranasal fixation or knots but thicker sections which help them self-retain within the nasolacrimal duct (Figure 8.8).

The success rate for adult silicone intubation for common canalicular obstruction is up to 75 per cent effective, and for nasolacrimal duct stenosis ranges between 25 and 68 per cent. Complications include punctal cheesewiring and tube prolapse at the medial canthus.

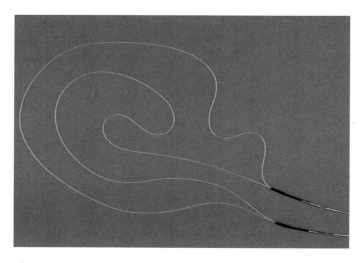

Figure 8.7

Double bicanalicular tubing (courtesy of Professor Hausler, Bern, Switzerland).

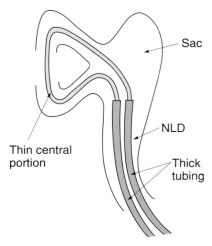

NLD = nasolacrimal duct

Figure 8.8

Diagram showing Nunchaku-style three-piece silicone tubing in place. The thicker silicone tubing makes this system self-retaining, without the need for knots or ties in the inferior meatus.

Balloon catheter dilation of the nasolacrimal duct (dacryoplasty)

There are two techniques for nasolacrimal duct dilation:

1. Transcanalicular insertion of deflated balloon for nasolacrimal duct dilation (dacryoplasty)
2. Transcanalicular guide wire and retrograde insertion of small bore angioplasty catheter into nasolacrimal duct, under fluoroscopic control.

Transcanalicular balloon catheter dilation

This uses the Lacricath system (Corinthian Medical Ltd, Sutton-in-Ashfield, Nottinghamshire, UK, or Atrion Medical Products, Birmingham, Alabama, USA), available in paediatric and adult sizes, 3 and 4 mm dilated diameters. There are 10 and 15 mm marks close to the balloon to help the surgeon know how far in the

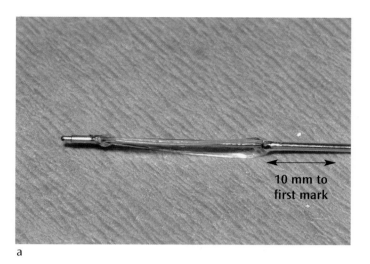

a

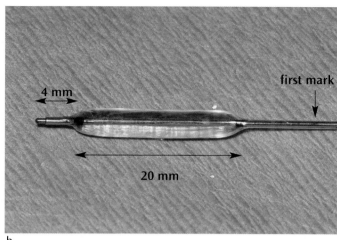

b

Figure 8.9

Lacricath balloon a) deflated and b) inflated with saline.

balloon has reached, assuming the canaliculi are approximately 10 mm long (Figure 8.9).

In adults, it is used in selected patients with functional epiphora from nasolacrimal duct stenosis (incomplete block confirmed on lacrimal scintigraphy) with subjective success rates of 60 per cent. Intubation may improve success rates. The balloon is also used to dilate the valve of Hasner in congenital nasolacrimal duct obstruction after failed probing, or in children over 2 years old.

Technique for adult balloon catheter dilation

Consent the patient for balloon catheter dilation with an option to proceed to endonasal DCR with tubes under local anaesthesia if indicated.

1. Use local anaesthetic regional infiltration to the anterior lacrimal crest and medial eyelids (as for endonasal DCR).
2. Decongest and anaesthetize the nasal mucosa, for example with cocaine 4 or 10% with adrenaline 1 in 20 000.
3. Syringe the lacrimal system to confirm incomplete block, as it may be several weeks since the lacrimal scintigraphy was done; if there is a complete block, consider proceeding to endonasal DCR.

4. Dilate either the upper or lower canaliculus well with the Nettleship dilator.
5. Place a Bowman probe size 1 in the canaliculus and advance it into the sac, respecting the natural curves in the canaliculus, particularly on entering the sac. Feel the medial wall of the sac (firm stop). Angulate the probe down towards the second molar tooth and probe the nasolacrimal duct in a posterior and lateral direction. If an obstruction is felt and the probe does not advance, abandon and convert to endonasal DCR or rebook the patient for later external DCR. If no obstruction is felt, repeat with size 2 Bowman probe, then the balloon catheter.
6. The assistant (often the anaesthetist) checks the pressure apparatus is functioning correctly. The large syringe is filled with saline, air in the tubes is evacuated and a three-way tap attached, more air is evacuated and then the balloon catheter is attached. Test inflating and deflating the balloon.
7. Coat the balloon with antibiotic ointment to ease its passage through the punctum. Pass the balloon exactly as the probe, until its tip emerges into the inferior meatus.
8. Start dilating the balloon when it is placed in the lower part of the duct and work upwards. Inflate the balloon to 9 bar for 90 s, repeating twice at each point (up to four points). Hold the wire still at the medial canthus to keep the balloon in place whilst

inflating it, otherwise it will slip towards a wider part of the duct (Figure 8.10). Deflate the balloon well between points. A small amount of bleeding will be visible at the punctum.

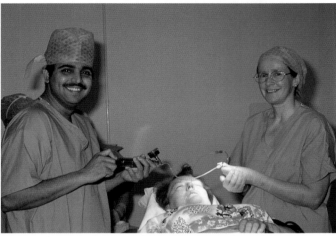

a

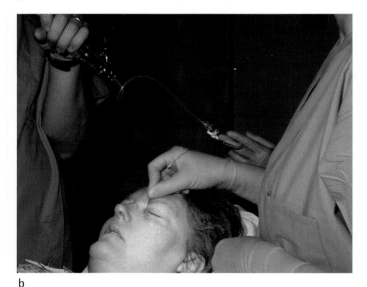

b

Figure 8.10

a) Patient having Lacricath balloon dilation. The assistant (left) holds the manometer and syringe whilst the surgeon (right) has placed the catheter in the lacrimal system and is holding the three-way tap prior to inflating the balloon.
b) Close-up, inflating the balloon. Note that a third person is holding the weight of the tubing and the surgeon is holding the catheter in place. Treatment is under local anaesthesia.

9. It is optional whether to intubate after dacryoplasty, and further studies are required to confirm the theoretical benefit. Results may be superior with intubation for up to 6 months.

TIP

The Bowman probe is 50 mm long and the maximum distance to the floor from the punctum is 40–45 mm, therefore you can estimate how far down the lacrimal system the probe has reached. Once it is in the inferior meatus, it can be seen endonasally.

Post-operative management

Give steroid antibiotic drops 2-hourly for 48 hours, then qds for 3 weeks. Apply topical antibiotics for 3 weeks. Some surgeons give oral antibiotics and steroids, but this is controversial because the benefits are not clear.

Review patient 6 weeks after dacryoplasty. If there are tubes, remove them 6–12 weeks post-operatively.

Assess the results based on the symptoms of epiphora, for example by using Munk's score or a lacrimal surgery subjective success assessment.

Munk's score of epiphora, scale 0–4:
0   No epiphora
1   Occasional epiphora requiring dabbing with a tissue or handkerchief less than twice a day
2   Epiphora requiring dabbing two to four times a day
3   Epiphora requiring dabbing five to ten times a day
4   Epiphora requiring dabbing more than ten times a day

Lacrimal surgery subjective success assessment:	
Success	No residual tearing at any time
Fair	Tearing outdoors only
Poor	Tearing persists indoors and outdoors

TIP

When assessing the subjective success of lacrimal surgery, remember that symptoms are naturally very much improved in summer (dry warm weather) compared to winter (windy cold weather).

Advantages and disadvantages of balloon dacryoplasty

Advantage:
- This is an easy local anaesthetic procedure suitable for elderly frail persons with mild epiphora from dacryostenosis (narrowing, but not complete block).

Disadvantages of balloon dacryoplasty:
- It gives only temporary symptomatic improvement
- There is a need to repeat balloon dacryoplasty or proceed to DCR within 6–48 months in about 50 per cent of cases owing to progressive disease.
- There is a high failure rate if you try and dilate complete nasolacrimal duct obstruction.

Transcanalicular guide wire and retrograde insertion of angioplasty catheter under fluoroscopic control

This is done jointly by the ophthalmologist and radiologist. The indications are incomplete or complete nasolacrimal duct stenosis. There are two techniques:
1. Retrograde angioplasty balloon catheter dilation
2. Retrograde angioplasty balloon catheter dilation and placement of metallic expandable stent.

Retrograde angioplasty balloon catheter dilation

1. Instil topical local anaesthesia to the surface of the eye and infiltrative anaesthesia to the medial eyelids and lacrimal fossa as for endonasal DCR.
2. Use topical nasal decongestant and local anaesthesia as for endonasal DCR.
3. Do an initial dacryocystography to confirm the location of duct stenosis.
4. Insert a 0.014 or 0.018 inch diameter guide wire through one punctum into the lacrimal system, and gently advance it through the nasolacrimal obstruction into the inferior meatus.
5. Under fluoroscopic guidance, insert a deflated 3–5 mm diameter, 3 or 4 cm long angioplasty balloon catheter retrogradely over the guide wire until it is within the point of maximum obstruction.
6. Inflate the balloon for 5 minutes with radiographic contrast medium, repeat with a larger sized balloon, and then remove the balloon transnasally.
7. With the guide wire in, repeat dacryocystography to confirm anatomical dilation. Repeat balloon dilation with 5 mm diameter balloon if there is still a stenosis. Remove the guide wire if well dilated.

Post-operative management

Apply guttae Maxitrol qds for 3 weeks. Review patient 6 weeks after dacryoplasty.

Complications/disadvantages

Complications include forming a false passage with the guide wire.

This is an expensive technique.

Retrograde angioplasty balloon catheter dilation and placement of metallic expandable stent

This is done as above, but with an additional step of inserting a metallic stent as used in cardiology. The stent expands to 4 mm in diameter and 20 mm in length.

Nasolacrimal duct stents

The initial expandable metallic stents have been replaced by a system using a polyurethane Song stent, without initial balloon dacryoplasty (Cook Group Company, Queensland, Australia). Indications for use include partial and complete nasolacrimal duct stenosis. Surgery is under local anaesthesia, usually with fluoroscopic guidance, with retrograde insertion of stent. The technical success rate is in the range of 96 per cent, but the clinical success rate is lower at 70–85 per cent. Long-term studies are still required.

The Song set consists of:
- A ball-tipped guide wire 0.018 inch in diameter
- A dark grey Teflon(tm) sleeve (stent introducer)
- A light grey pusher catheter (injector)
- A white polyurethane lacrimal stent (mushroom head).

The head of the stent is 5–6 mm in diameter when expanded, and its length is 6–9 mm. The body is 35 mm long (Figures 8.11, 8.12).

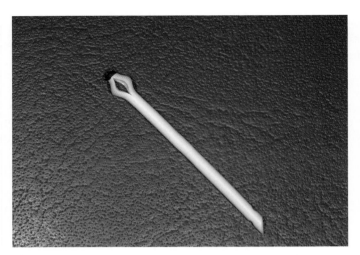

Figure 8.11
Song stent with expanded head.

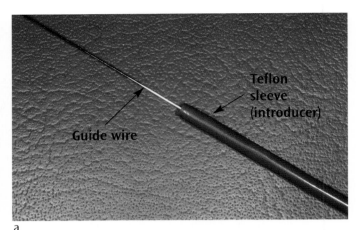

a

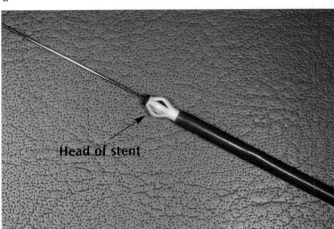

b

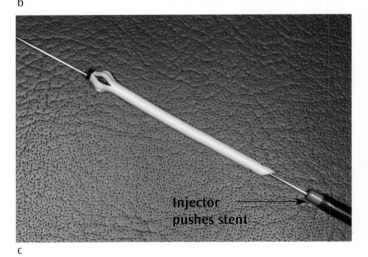

c

Procedure:

1. Introduce either a guide wire or a Ritleng introducer via the lower or upper punctum into the lacrimal system.
2. Introduce the grey Teflon sleeve in a retrograde direction up the guide wire. The sleeve contains the expandable 'mushroom'-tipped stent and injector.
3. Advance the stent into the nasolacrimal duct until correctly positioned.
4. Withdraw the sleeve and injector downwards, and then the wire upwards.

Complications

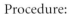

● Canalicular stenosis
● Acute dacryocystitis.

TIP

Inserting the guide wire via the lower punctum risks damaging the lower canaliculus with resultant stenosis. Some surgeons prefer the upper punctum.

Figure 8.12

a) Guide wire (left) and grey sleeve stent introducer (right).
b) Mushroom head of stent emerging from introducer. The mushroom sits in the lower part of the lacrimal sac.
c) Stent fully injected. The light grey injector tube is just visible within the darker introducer tube.

Bibliography

Botulinum toxin:

Hofman, R. J. (2000). Treatment of Frey's syndrome (gustatory sweating) and 'crocodile tears' (gustatory epiphora) with purified botulinum toxin. *Ophthal. Plast. Reconstr. Surg.*, 16, 289–91.

Riemann, R., Pfennigsdorf, S., Rieman, E. and Naumann, M. (1999). Successful treatment of crocodile tears by injection of botulinum toxin into the lacrimal gland. *Ophthalmology*, 106, 2322–4.

Silicone plugs:

Akova, Y. A., Demirhan, B., Cakmakci, S. and Aydin, P. (1999). Pyogenic granuloma: a rare complication of silicone punctal plugs. *Ophthal. Surg. Lasers*, 30, 584–5.

Glatt, H. J. (1992). Failure of collagen plugs to predict epiphora after permanent punctal occlusion. *Ophthal. Surg.*, 23, 292–3.

Transcanalicular endoscopy, canaliculoplasty and DCR:

Dalez, D. and Lemagne, J. M. (1996). Transcanicular dacryocystorhinostomy by pulse holmium-YAG laser. *Bull. Soc. Belge. Ophthalmol.*, 263, 139–40 (French).

Dutton, J. J. and Holck, D. E. (1996). Holmium laser canaliculoplasty. *Ophthal. Plast. Reconstr. Surg.*, 12, 211–17.

Eloy, P., Trussart, C., Jouzdani, E. *et al.* (2000). Transcanalicular diode laser-assisted dacryocystorhinostomy. *Acta Otorhinolaryngol. Belg.*, 54, 157–63.

Kuchar, A., Novak, P., Pieh, S. *et al.* (1999). Endoscopic laser recanalisation of presaccal canalicular obstruction. *Br. J. Ophthalmol.*, 83, 443–7.

Muellner, K. and Wolf, G. (1999). Endoscopic treatment of lacrimal duct stenosis using a KTP laser – report of initial experiences (in German). *Klin. Monatsbl. Augenheilkd*, 205, 28–32.

Muellner, K., Bodner, E. and Mannor, G. E. (1999). Endoscopy of the lacrimal system. *Br. J. Ophthalmol.*, 83, 949–52.

Muellner, K., Bodner, E., Mannor, G. E. *et al.* (2000). Endolacrimal laser assisted lacrimal surgery. *Br. J. Ophthalmol.*, 84, 16–18.

Patel, B. C., Phillips, B., McLeish, W. M., Flaherty, P. and Anderson, R. L. (1997). Transcanicular neodymium:YAG laser for revision of dacryocystorhinostomy. *Ophthalmology*, 104, 1191–7.

Piaton, J. M., Limon, S., Ounnan, N. and Keller, P. (1994). Transcanicular endodacryocystorhinostomy using neodymium:YAG laser. *J. Fr. Ophthalmol.*, 17, 555–67 (French).

Rosen, N., Barak, A. and Rosner, M. (1997). Transcanicular dacryocystorhinostomy. *Ophthalmic Surg. Lasers*, 28, 723–6.

Nasolacrimal intubation:

Beigi, B. and O'Keefe, M. (1993). Results of Crawford tube intubation in children. *Acta Ophthalmol. (Copenhagen)*, 71, 405–7.

Fulcher, T., O'Connor, M. and Moriaty, P. (1998). Nasolacrimal intubation in adults. *Br. J. Ophthalmol.*, 82, 1039–41.

Kurihashi, K. (1994). A new bicanalicular intubation method. Direct silicone intubation (DSI). *Orbit.*, 13, 11–15.

Balloon dilation and stents:

Becker, B. B., Berry, F. D. and Koller, H. (1996). Balloon catheter dilation for treatment of congenital nasolacrimal duct obstruction. *Am. J. Ophthalmol.*, 121, 304–9.

Ilgit, E. T., Yuksel, D., Unal, M. *et al.* (1995). Transluminal balloon dilatation of the lacrimal drainage system for the treatment of epiphora. *Am. J. Radiol.*, 165, 1517–24.

Lee, S. L., Jung, G., Oum, B. S. *et al.* (2000). Clinical efficacy of the polyurethane stent without fluoroscopic guidance in the treatment of nasolacrimal duct obstruction. *Ophthalmology*, 107, 1666–70.

Munk, P. L., Lin, D. T. C. and Morris, D. C. (1990). Epiphora: treatment by means of dacryoplasty with balloon dilation of the nasolacrimal drainage apparatus. *Radiology*, 177, 687–90.

Perry, J. D., Maus, M., Nowinski, T. S. and Penne, R. B. 1998). Balloon catheter dilation for the treatment of adults with partial nasolacrimal duct obstruction: a preliminary report. *Am. J. Ophthalmol.*, 126, 811–16.

Song, H., Ahn, H., Park, C. *et al.* (1993). Complete obstruction of the nasolacrimal system. Part I, Treatment with balloon dilation; Part II, Treatment with expandable metallic stents. *Radiology*, 186, 367–71 and 372–6.

Yazici, Z., Yazici, B., Parlak, M. *et al.* (1999). Treatment of obstructive epiphora in adults by balloon dacryoplasty. *Br. J. Ophthalmol.*, 83, 692–6.

Index